D1677839

# von Willebrand Disease and von Willebrand Factor

## Current Aspects of Diagnosis and Treatment

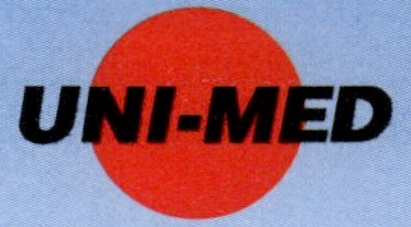


UNI-MED Verlag AG
Bremen - London - Boston

Prof. Dr Reinhard Schneppenheim
University Medical Center Hamburg-Eppendorf
Dept. of Pediatric Hematology and Oncology
Martinistr. 52
20246 Hamburg
Germany

Prof. Dr Ulrich Budde
AescuLabor Hamburg
Haferweg 36
22769 Hamburg
Germany

**Schneppenheim, Reinhard:**
von Willebrand Disease and von Willebrand Factor - Current Aspects of Diagnosis and Treatment/
Reinhard Schneppenheim and Ulrich Budde.-
1. Auflage - Bremen: UNI-MED, 2008
(UNI-MED SCIENCE)
ISBN 978-3-8374-1009-9
ISBN 978-1-84815-131-4



Printed in Europe

# *MEDICINE - STATE OF THE ART*

UNI-MED Verlag AG, one of the leading medical publishing companies in Germany, presents its highly successful series of scientific textbooks, covering all medical subjects. The authors are specialists in their fields and present the topics precisely, comprehensively, and with the facility of quick reference in mind. The books will be most useful for all doctors who wish to keep up to date with the latest developments in medicine.

# Preface

Writing the preface to a scientific publication, particularly when the work originates from a couple of esteemed colleagues and good friends, may be easy and difficult at the same time. What is a preface supposed to be, after all? Should it contain just words of praise (the easy part) to convince a potential reader, or a critical review (the difficult part) to provide a perspective on how the subject material is treated in the text? I accepted my task because I was confident that the authors wanted me to do both, in other words they were asking for an honest introduction to their work for its potential audience. Here are eighty plus pages on von Willebrand disease and von Willebrand factor, going from historical introductory notes to a presentation of the current understanding of von Willebrand factor structure and function to an extensive excursus on the pathogenesis, classification, diagnosis and treatment of von Willebrand disease, including congenital and acquired forms. One final chapter is dedicated to thrombotic thrombocytopenic purpura, a well distinct syndrome but linked to von Willebrand disease through the common pathogenetic involvement of von Willebrand factor. The topics addressed in the monograph are undoubtedly relevant, as von Willebrand disease is one of the most common congenital bleeding disorders, sometimes difficult to diagnose and treat properly, and most physicians will likely encounter one such patient in the course of their professional life. Acquired forms are supposedly less common, but are likely underdiagnosed. Thrombotic thrombocytopenic purpura, congenital or acquired, is rare, but usually fatal if not properly diagnosed and managed. This monograph can put the reader on the right track to acquire a general understanding of the clinical and laboratory problems at hand, while also representing a useful reference text to consult for detailed information and support when dealing with a suspected case. The authors' direct and intimate knowledge of the topics they address transpires clearly through the lines, particularly in the chapters dealing with molecular genetics and laboratory tests. The monograph is well balanced, with good pictures and clear tables and schemes. This work is addressed to an audience not necessarily consisting of specialists in thrombosis and hemostasis, thus it has to be exhaustive but cannot go to the core of current basic research aimed at finding the answers to still unsolved questions relevant for a better understanding of von Willebrand disease and von Willebrand factor. For that, interested readers will have to use more specific reviews and original publications. But for all those interested in knowing how von Willebrand disease is diagnosed and treated, as well as understanding the pathogenesis of the diseases, this monograph will provide the state-of-the art picture in 2008.

*La Jolla, California, July 2008* *Zaverio M. Ruggeri*

# Contents

# History

# 1. History

von Willebrand disease (VWD) was first described in 1926 in Helsinki by Erik Adolf von Willebrand, a Finnish general physician, using the example of a family from the island of Föglö in the Åland archipelago in the Baltic Sea (☞ Figure 1.1). von Willebrand called the condition hereditary pseudohemophilia. This was in reference to the bleeding tendency in common with hemophilia albeit with a usually normal clotting time, but, in contrast to hemophilia, with a prolonged bleeding time. Moreover, in contrast to hemophilia, females were also affected by the bleeding tendency. Indeed, since females appeared to be even more affected by the bleeding tendency, von Willebrand described the inheritance as sex-associated and dominant.

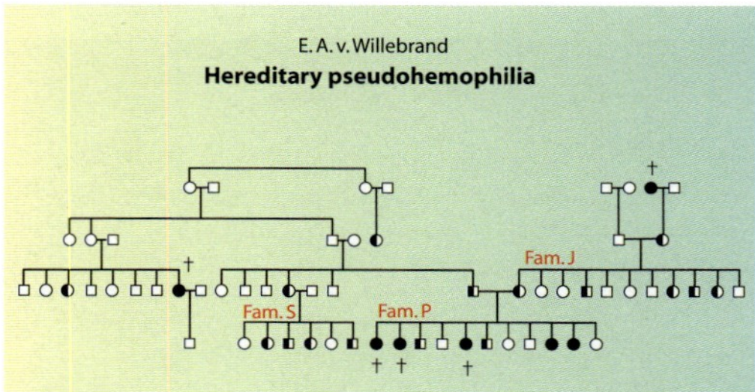


***Figure 1.1:*** Family from the Åland islands. + = died from hemorrhage (Hereditary pseudohemophilia. E. A. v. Willebrand, Finska Läkaresällskapets Handlingar Vol. LXVII, No. 2, 1926).

The more severe course described in females among the family members was in many cases attributed to "female-specific" types of bleeding, such as prolonged, severe menstrual bleeding and hemorrhage after labor. Some girls and women in this family had bled to death. In his paper, von Willebrand also reported the literature known up to that point. It was clear from this that so-called "female hemophilia" had also previously been reported. In particular, the Giessen-based gynecologist Kehrer had described such cases in great detail in his monograph that appeared in 1876, such as the medical history of a woman who, after three miscarriages with subsequent severe bleeding complications, had eventually bled to death a month after her fourth miscarriage. Her father had suffered from severe nose bleeds (☞ Figure 1.2).

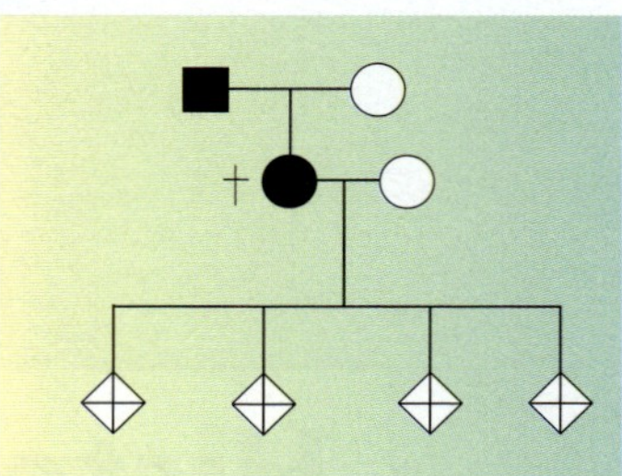

***Figure 1.2:*** Pedigree of a family with "female hemophilia" described by Kehrer. All pregnancies of the index patient ended in miscarriages, and she bled to death at the time of her last one (Hemophilia in the female sex. F.A. Kehrer, Archiv für Gynäkologie, Vol. X No. 2, p. 14-237).

Another female patient whose father suffered frequent nose bleeds also bled to death two months after the birth of her third child. von Willebrand also summarized this case and others in his original paper and discussed them in relation to the family that he himself had studied. It was thus thanks to him that the disease that would later bear his name came to be differentiated from hemophilia as an entity in itself.

In 1933, further details of this new blood disease were published in a joint study in conjunction with the Leipzig hematologist Jürgens. Thus, among other things, a tendency towards decreased platelet aggregation was discovered in some of these patients. The evaluation of the bleeding tendency in regard to this as a primary platelet disorder led to the term "von Willebrand-Jürgens thrombopathy". It is due to this study that the term "von Willebrand-Jürgens syndrome" is still in use today in German. The term von Willebrand disease (VWD) is the international name now generally used.

In the 1940s, there were more and more reports of cases of hemorrhagic diseases with the main symptoms being a prolonged bleeding time and decreased capillary resistance in the presence of a normal platelet count and coagulation. The primary defect was considered to be a vasculopathy, since some patients were also found to have capillary abnormalities. These findings led to the terms "vascular hemophilia" or "angiohemophilia."

In 1953, Alexander and Goldstein noted an association between factor VIII (FVIII) and a prolonged bleeding time in patients with VWD. In 1959, Nilsson, and colleagues showed that infusion of Cohn's fraction I-0 shortened the bleeding time and that the half-life of FVIII in patients with VWD after infusion of Cohn's fraction I-0 was longer than in patients with hemophilia. The increase in FVIII after infusion continued for several hours, in complete contrast to the rapid rise after replacement in patients with hemophilia A. Furthermore, patients were even found to have an unexpected increase in FVIII if they were transfused with plasma from patients with hemophilia A. In contrast, the infusion of plasma from patients with VWD did not result in a rise in FVIII in patients with hemophilia A. These observations prompted Nilsson and colleagues to postulate for the first time a plasma factor that corrected the bleeding time, which clearly had to be different from FVIII.

In 1971, Zimmermann and colleagues were the first to immunologically identify this new factor, which is today called von Willebrand factor (VWF) and initially called it FVIII-associated antigen because of its association with FVIII. Biochemical and immunological studies subsequently clearly showed that FVIII and VWF are the product of different genes on different chromosomes and that deficiency or qualitative defects of these caused different hemorrhagic diseases, namely, hemophilia A and VWD.

The gene sequence coding for VWF was published simultaneously by several groups in 1985. The molecular diagnosis that became possible as a result of this has made an enormous contribution to explaining the role of VWF, not just in bleeding events but also in relation to thrombosis. The different early clinical and experimental observations, which were even accompanied by differentiation into different clinical pictures and led to lasting scientific controversy, found reconciliation with the discovery of the multifactorial nature of VWF and are, as we now know, an expression of the marked heterogeneity of VWD. A special illustration of this is the identification of an FVIII-binding domain of VWF. Defects of this domain as a result of mutations lead to isolated FVIII deficiency, which initially cannot be differentiated from hemophilia A. The term hereditary "pseudohemophilia" initially coined by E. A. von Willebrand took on special topicality as a result of these discoveries, and this term is indeed justified in the true sense at least for a small number of patients with VWD.

# Clinical Symptoms and Genetics

# 2. Clinical Symptoms and Genetics

## 2.1. Clinical symptoms of von Willebrand disease (VWD)

Because of its multifunctional nature, very different defects of VWF may arise and thus lead to clinically different manifestations of the bleeding tendency. In purely quantitative defects of VWF, a similar reduction in VWF:Ag and function may be expected. In contrast, qualitative defects may affect specific functions of VWF without the VWF:Ag level being reduced. In general, therefore, combinations of disorders of primary and secondary hemostasis (type 1, type 3 VWD), isolated disorders of primary hemostasis (e.g. type 2A) and isolated disorders of secondary hemostasis (type 2N) are seen.

The main symptom of classic VWD is prolonged mucosal bleeding (☞ Figure 2.1).

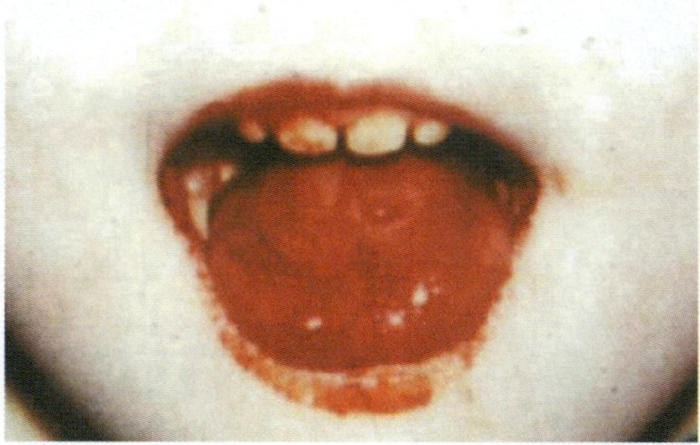

***Figure 2.1:*** Oozing hemorrhage from the mouth of a 4-year-old girl with type 3 VWD . The source of bleeding could not be localized. The hemoglobin fell to 5 g/dL.

This is seen as bleeding during teething and after tonsillectomy, adenotomy and tooth extraction. Indeed, it is during operations in the mucosal region that surprising bleeding episodes may occur in a patient who previously had been unremarkable in relation to a bleeding diathesis. Women additionally have symptoms from prolonged and more severe menstrual bleeding and postnatal hemorrhage. Bleeding from the gastrointestinal tract and the urogenital system also occurs. Nose bleeds and superficial hematomas are very common (☞ Table 2.1).

| | Italy only VWD (n=1,286) | | | Scandinavia | |
|---|---|---|---|---|---|
| | Type 1 n=944 | Type 2 n=268 | Type 3 n=74 | VWD n=264 | Normal n=500 |
| Epistaxis | 56 | 63 | 74 | 62 | 5 |
| Menorrhagia | 31 | 32 | 32 | 60 | 25 |
| Bleeding after tooth extraction | 31 | 39 | 53 | 51 | 5 |
| Hematomas | 14 | 19 | 31 | 49 | 12 |
| Bleeding from small wounds | 36 | 40 | 50 | 36 | 0.2 |
| Mucosal bleeding | 30 | 37 | 48 | 35 | 7 |
| Postoperative bleeding | 20 | 23 | 41 | 28 | 1 |
| Postpartum bleeding | 17 | 18 | 26 | 23 | 19 |
| Gastrointestinal bleeding | 5 | 11 | 18 | 14 | 1 |
| Bleeding into joints | 2 | 5 | 42 | 8 | 0 |
| Hematuria | 2 | 4 | 11 | 7 | 1 |
| Intracerebral hemorrhage | 0.5 | 0.3 | 8 | Not reported | 0 |

***Table 2.1:*** Bleeding symptoms (%) in patients with VWD and normal individuals, based on Rodeghiero and Castaman 2001, with permission.

Bleeding into muscles and joints, as occurs in hemophilia, is rare however, is usually associated with severe VWD or VWD 2N with greatly reduced FVIII, and indicates an additional or isolated disorder of secondary hemostasis. In a retrospective study undertaken by us, the rate of bleeding into joints was 76% in 32 patients with severe type 3 VWD, while the rate of bleeding into muscles was 24%. Figure 2.2 shows the most common symptoms of bleeding in severe type 3 VWD.

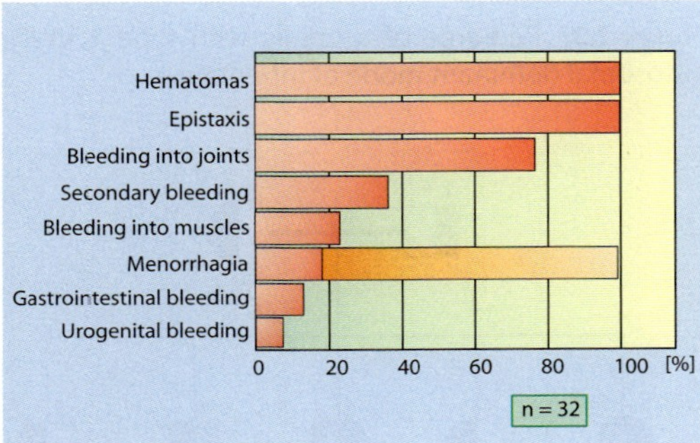


***Figure 2.2:*** Spectrum of bleeding symptoms in severe type 3 VWD. All 6 female patients (100%) after the menarche had severe menorrhagia.

A particular problem is bleeding during menstruation or postpartum. Studies give the prevalence of VWD in women with menorrhagia as 7-20%. Conversely, it has been shown that depending on the severity, 74% to 100% of women with VWD have menorrhagia. In one population that was studied, 66% had type 1 VWD. This means that even in mild VWD, the majority of women have menorrhagia. It is often difficult in this situation to elicit menorrhagia from the history. The affected women often do not know that they have heavy bleeding. In principle, female patients with VWD 3 have menorrhagia. If in a family the mothers are also affected, which is not uncommon given the dominant mode of inheritance, comparison with the mother is not much help either. Thus, patients occasionally present with marked iron deficiency anemia and hemoglobin levels <6 g/dL and who, on questioning, report menstrual bleeding for more than 14 days, without regarding this as being excessive. Even today, isolated cases of deaths resulting from menstrual bleeding that cannot be stopped are reported. The rate of hysterectomies because of menorrhagia has been reported as 23% in women with type 2 or 3 VWD. In patients with type 1 VWD, rates of 8-10% are reported. In most cases that have been described in detail, the diagnosis of VWD was made after hysterectomy. As a rough guide to assess the amount of menstrual bleeding, questions should be asked about the duration, how often pads or tampons have to be changed and to what extent they are blood-soaked. If the suspected menorrhagia is confirmed, diagnostic clotting tests should always be undertaken.

To assess the diagnostic probability of VWD, questionaires have been designed that result in a bleeding score. A very comprehensive questionaire that also satisfies scientific requirements is currently recommended by the International Society of Thrombosis and Haemaostasis (☞ ISTH URL: http://www.med.unc.edu/isth/ssc/collaboration/Bleeding_Type1_VWD.pdf). The questionaire also allows negative scores in cases of non-bleeding after adequate challenge (e.g. non-bleeding after tonsillectomy or after 2 births).

With the exception of patients with severe VWD 3, a rise in the VWF:Ag will be found in virtually all women during the course of pregnancy. However, the sharpest increase is not found until the third trimester. In most cases, this is accompanied by an improvement in hemostasis, so the bleeding tendency decreases. Thus, many births in women with VWD take place without major blood loss. However, there are ever more examples of patients either with severe VWD or with qualitative defects of VWF in whom birth is accompanied by uncontrollable postpartum hemorrhage thus leading to hysterectomy often without awareness of the underlying diagnosis. Women with type 2B VWD are a special group. In these patients, depending on the rise in the VWF:Ag there may be a more or less severe decrease in the functionally most important high molecular weight VWF multimers and accompanying thrombocytopenia with an increased bleeding tendency (☞ type 2B VWD for the pathogenetic mechanism). In patients with milder forms of VWD, hemorrhagic complications do not usually occur until the puerperal period. After birth, the VWF:Ag decreases again and the puerperal flow may again appear bloody if adequate hemostasis is no longer guaranteed.

The type of bleeding, bleeding frequency and clinical severity are also dependent on other modulating diseases such as angiodysplasia, telangiectasia and cardiac defects. It was recently shown that polymorphism in the collagen receptor for platelets (GPIa/IIa) modulates the expression of this receptor 10-fold and that the bleeding tendency in patients with type 1 VWD increases greatly if there is low expression of the receptor.

## 2.2. Clinical genetics of VWD

The pedigree of the original family from the Åaland islands did not allow any clear mode of inheritance of VWD to be identified. von Willebrand assumed an autosomal mode of inheritance, albeit with an association with sex. It was noted that women in particular were especially affected clinically by the bleeding tendency. This was very probably because of the marked bleeding during menstruation and labor. Some girls and women in this family died as a result of exsanguination. From molecular genetic investigations of the descendants of the Åaland family, we now know that the severe outcomes probably followed an autosomal recessive mode of inheritance. Today, a clear distinction can be made between autosomal recessive and autosomal dominant inheritance of VWD. Type 1 VWD, which tends to have mild symptoms, has a dominant mode of inheritance with affected individuals in successive generations (☞ Figure 2.3), while severe type 3 VWD has a recessive mode of inheritance and is found more often in societies with consanguineous marriages (☞ Figure 2.4). Speculation as to whether severe type 3 VWD is caused by inheritance of two type 1 VWD defects has been confirmed only in exceptional cases. Based on recent findings from molecular diagnostic techniques, type 1 appears to be a group in its own right with dominant negative mutations. In fact, heterozygous gene carriers of a type 3 defect may be completely unremarkable clinically and on laboratory investigation.

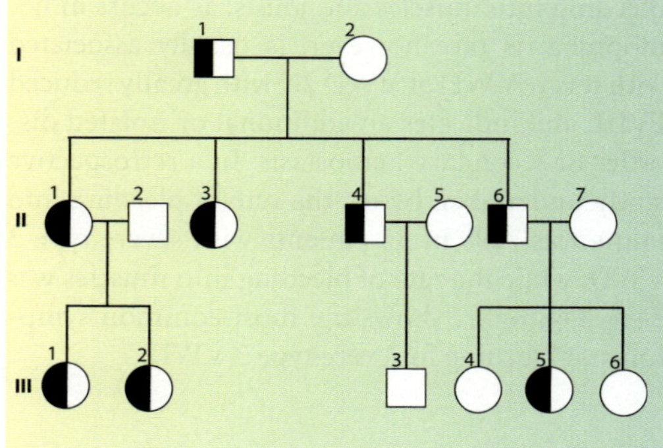


***Figure 2.3:*** Pedigree of a family with type 1 VWD: autosomal dominant mode of inheritance.

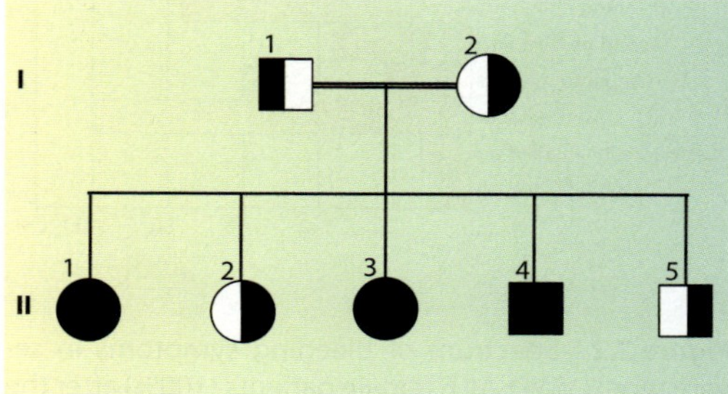


***Figure 2.4:*** Pedigree of a family with severe type 3 VWD: autosomal recessive mode of inheritance in consanguinity.

Type 2 VWD shows, in most cases, dominant inheritance (☞ Figure 2.5). Given the structure of VWF, which consists of multimers of the same subunits, the dominant negative effect of only one qualitatively defective allele on the whole molecule is easily understood. This has an effect principally on the processes of dimerization, multimerization, intracellular transport, sensitivity to ADAMTS13-mediated proteolysis (☞ Chapt. 8.) and functionally in relation to the affinity for the platelet GP Ib. In contrast, a purely quantitative defect of only one allele appears to be insufficient for VWD, since this is unable to influence the structure of VWF.

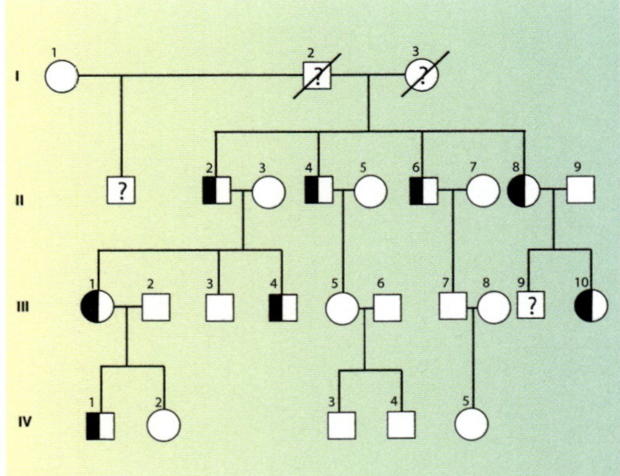


***Figure 2.5:*** Pedigree of a family with type 2A VWD: autosomal dominant mode of inheritance.

Two rare subtypes of VWD type 2 do, however, show recessive inheritance. These include type 2N VWD with disturbed FVIII-binding capacity of VWF, which presents like hemophilia (☞ Figure 2.6).

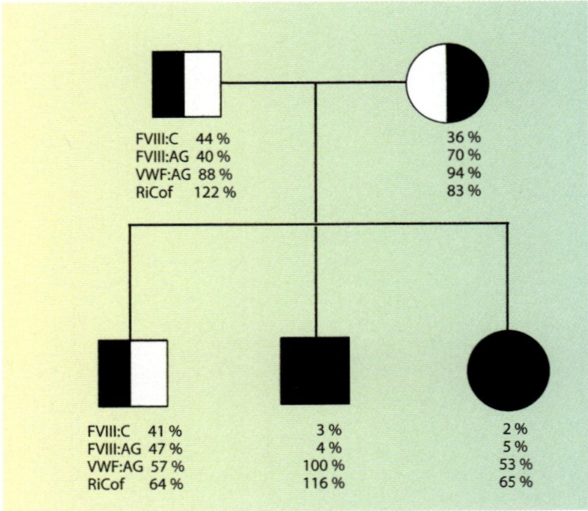


***Figure 2.6:*** Pedigree of a family with type 2N VWD: autosomal recessive mode of inheritance. Phenotype as in hemophilia A.

Here, the combination of two FVIII binding defects or a FVIII binding defect with a quantitative defect (e.g. type 3 defect) are possible. Only in the case of the latter is a low VWF detectable. The second example concerns the VWD subtype 2A, subgroup IIC. The defects are localized in the D1 and/or D2 domain of the VWF propeptide. This propeptide is cleaved by proteolysis, but initially functions normally as a disulfide isomerase in disulfide bond formation of VWF dimers at the aminoterminal end resulting in multimerization. Enzyme activity of the propeptide half that of normal appears to be sufficient for this so only defects of both alleles, i.e. homozygous or compound heterozygous mutations can reduce multimerization and thus explain the occurrence of VWD 2A subgroup IIC and the recessive inheritance (☞ Figure 2.7).

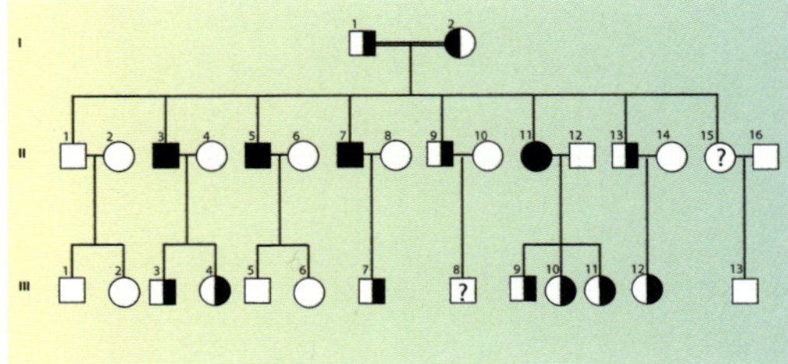


***Figure 2.7:*** Pedigree of a family with VWD type 2A subgroup IIC: autosomal recessive mode of inheritance in consanguinity.

The large number of different quantitative, structural and functional defects of VWF allows many combination possibilities and provides some insight into the clinical and genetic heterogeneity of VWD.

# von Willebrand Factor (VWF)

# 3. von Willebrand Factor (VWF)

## 3.1. Biosynthesis

von Willebrand factor (VWF) is synthesized in endothelial cells and megakaryocytes. The fact that it is limited to these cell types means it is a specific marker for the identification of endothelial cells in histological sections and a megakaryocyte marker, e.g. for the diagnosis of megakayrocyte leukemia.

The primary product consists of a pre-pro-VWF, a monomer of 2,813 amino acids and a molecular weight of 360 kilodalton (kd). This monomer undergoes complex biochemical and structural modifications. These result in multimers with the same composition, but, depending on the number of monomers, they have a different size of between 500-20,000 kd (☞ Figure 3.1).

The VWF is initially glycosylated, sulfated and dimerized in the endoplasmic reticulum via disulfide bonds on the carboxyterminal end of the protein, the cystine knot-like domain (CK domain). Mutations in this region of VWF lead to disordered dimerization and thus to a special form of VWD 2A, subtype IID. The identification of these mutations in relation to the observed phenotype has confirmed the previous experimental and theoretical considerations of VWF biosynthesis.

The VWF propeptide of 763 amino acids, which is subsequently split, is necessary for further polymerization of the VWF dimers, this time at the aminoterminal end. For this, it has amino acid consensus sequences (CGLC) in the D1 and D2 domain identical to disulfide isomerase that are thought to be essential for multimerization. Changes in these consensus sequences and mutations in proximity to them lead to defects of multimerization (☞ Chapt. 4.2.3.2.). Mutations in the D3 domain, which principally concern cysteine residues, have similar consequences. A CGLC sequence is also found in the D3 domain; mutagenesis of this sequence leads to impaired multimerization. A further CGLC sequence in the D4 domain does not appear to have any relevance to multimerization. Following further polymerization in the Golgi and post-Golgi compartment, VWF achieves its enormous size of 20,000 kd (☞ Figure 3.2).

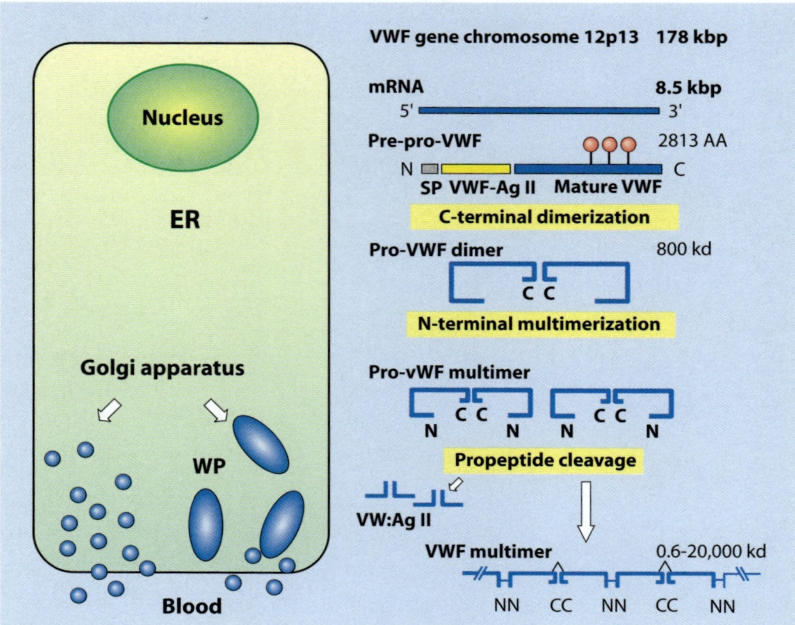


***Figure 3.1:*** Biosynthesis of VWF in the endothelial cell. ER = endoplasmatic reticulum; WP = Weibel-Palade bodies.

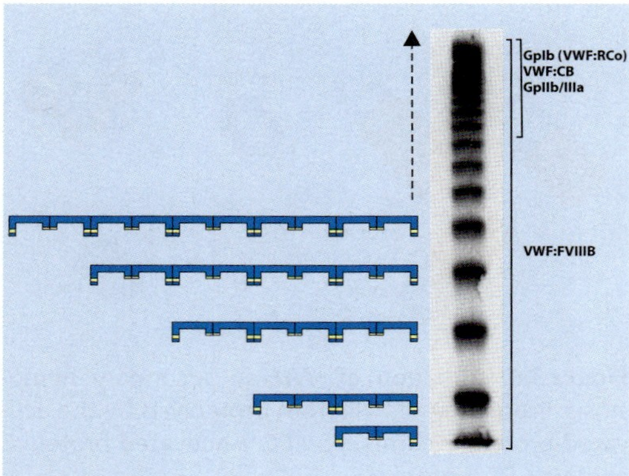


***Figure 3.2:*** Dimerization and multimerization of VWF and corresponding bands in SDS agarose gel electrophoresis.

The building blocks of multimerization are disulfide bonds between several cysteines in the D3 domain of VWF, which have not yet been fully identified. The recent observation that several mutations in this region, predominantly affecting cysteine residues, result in a disturbance of multimerization is interesting. Here, too, observations in patients have thus contributed to explaining and confirming essential steps in the post-translational biosynthesis of VWF. VWF is either constitutively released into plasma or initially stored in so-called Weibel-Palade bodies and released in response to an appropriate signal (e.g. thrombin, plasmin, fibrin). This release may also occur through the vasopressin analogue DDAVP (☞ Figure 3.3).

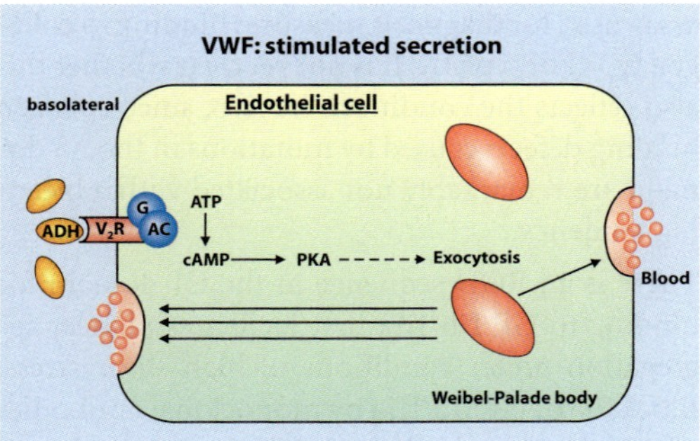


***Figure 3.3:*** Hypothetical signaling chain for VWF release into the blood and subendothelium following DDAVP, mediated by vasopressin receptor 2 (V2R), G-protein (G), adenylate cyclase (AC) and protein kinase A (PKA).

VWF is the largest soluble protein in humans with a plasma concentration of ca. 10 µg/mL. Its size and thus its biological activity are regulated by a specific VWF cleaving protease (VWF-CP), a metalloprotease (ADAMTS13), which splits VWF between tyrosine 1605 and methionine 1606 in the A2 domain (☞ Figure 3.4).

## 3.2. Structure-function relationships

VWF contains several copies of functional domains that possess specific binding sites for soluble and cellular components. These include binding sites for FVIII, collagen, heparin and platelet glycoproteins GP Ib and GP IIb/IIIa (☞ Figure 3.4).

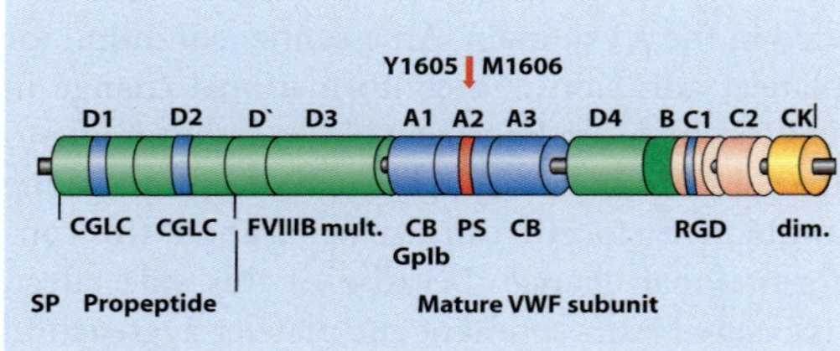


***Figure 3.4:*** Structure of the VWF monomer. The different domains with different functional regions are shown. CGLC disulfide disomerase consensus sequence, FVIIIB = FVIII binding region, mult. = multimerization region, CB = collagen binding region, GP Ib = binding region for GP Ib, PS = proteolytic cleavage site of VWF for ADAMTS13 in the A2 domain between tyrosine1605 and methionine 1606, RGD = binding sequence for GP IIb/IIIa, dim. = dimerization region (CK domain), SP = signal peptide.

Under conditions of high shear stress, i.e. in the arterial system and capillary region, VWF facilitates the adhesion of platelets to the subendothelium and also promotes platelet aggregation. The initially reversible adhesion of platelets to the injured or exposed subendothelium is mediated by the interaction between VWF and subendothelial components such as collagen. During this process, VWF experiences structural modifications that promote its interactions with GP Ib. These initial events lead to exposure of the platelet GP IIb/IIIa complexes, which in turn are essential for irreversible binding to the subendothelium, platelet aggregation and thrombus formation (☞ Figure 3.5).

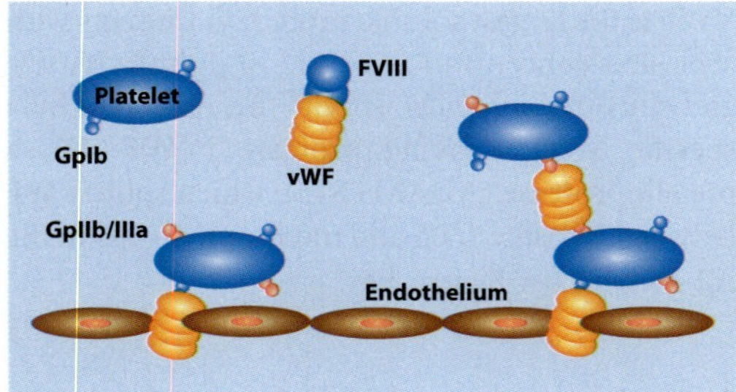


***Figure 3.5:*** Function of VWF in primary hemostasis.

The VWF multimers with the highest molecular weight are the most effective multimers in primary hemostasis. This accounts for the special importance of high-molecular-weight VWF, including in plasma concentrates. Selective absence of these large multimers leads to specific forms of VWD, type 2A and type 2B (☞ Chapt. 4.).

The VWF binding region for platelet GP Ib is situated in the A1 domain. An essential condition for platelet adhesion is a conformational change in VWF, which can be triggered through binding to the subendothelium and by high shear forces. The antibiotic ristocetin can also bring about this conformational change. Because of this side effect, associated with spontaneous platelet aggregation and thrombocytopenia, ristocetin is no longer used as a drug, but is still used in the diagnosis of von Willebrand disease (VWD) in the assay of the ristocetin cofactor (VWF:RCo). Spontaneous platelet aggregation is also seen in patients with mutations of the A1 domain. These mutations, which are located in a specific region of the A1 domain, lead to increased affinity of VWF for GP Ib and correlate with type 2B VWD (☞ Chapt. 4.).

The binding of FVIII is the second important function of VWF (☞ Figure 3.6) and does not depend on the size of the VWF multimers. FVIII that is bound to VWF is relatively protected against proteolytic attack by the protein C complex and possibly other proteases.

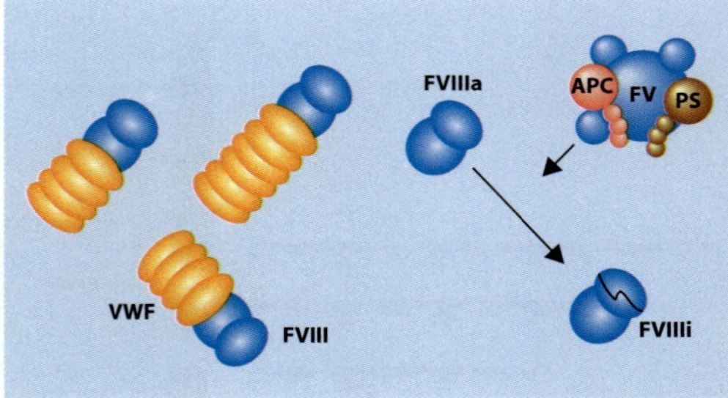


***Figure 3.6:*** Function of VWF in secondary hemostasis. Protection of FVIII from proteolysis by the activated protein C complex. APC = activated protein C complex, PS = protein S.

Absence of this protection in the case of VWF deficiency or a functional defect in the FVIII binding region of VWF is correlated with marked FVIII deficiency of between 1-9%, with a median of 3%. Only in these instances is there a significant defect of secondary hemostasis and clinical symptoms that are also seen in hemophilia, such as bleeding into muscles and joints.

Other binding regions exist for collagen, heparin and GP IIb/IIIa. The collagen binding of VWF is considered to be an important function in primary hemostasis. It is believed to be responsible for anchoring of VWF in the subendothelium, through which adhesion of platelets is mediated. Two collagen binding regions, one in the A1 domain and one in the A3 domain have so far been described. The A3 domain is the main binding site for collagen type I and type III, while the A1 domain is the binding site for collagen type VI. The collagen binding assay used for diagnosis measures binding to collagen type I or type III. It is not yet clear whether this also reflects the conditions in vivo, since collagen binding defects caused by mutations in the A3 domain are remarkably not associated with a bleeding tendency.

There is an RGD sequence in the C1 domain for binding to GP IIb/IIIa that facilitates platelet aggregation under conditions of high shear stress. Blockade of GP IIb/IIIa by monoclonal antibodies is used therapeutically for inhibition of platelet aggregation.

## 3.3. Molecular genetics

The gene for VWF is situated on the distal end of the short arm of chromosome 12 (12p13.3). It consists of 178 kilobases (kb), spread over 52 exons and 51 introns. The coding sequence contains 8,439 nucleotides (nt) for 2,813 amino acids. The gene contains several repeating homologous regions that have arisen through gene replication and fusion during evolution (☞ Figure 3.4). Analysis of the VWF gene is complicated by the existence of a pseudogene on chromosome 22. This is 97% homologous with exons 24-34 of the actual gene. The pseudogene makes molecular diagnostics through PCR difficult. For specific amplification, primers must be selected that differentiate between the gene and the pseudogene.

### Quantitative defects

The first gene defects were described in severe type 3 VWD. Before the advent of PCR, initially only large, mostly complete homozygous deletions of the gene were identified using the Southern blot technique. After the invention of PCR by Kary Mullis, point mutations were also easily identified. In type 3 VWD, small deletions are mainly found, which lead to shifting of the reading frame and nonsense mutations resulting in unstable RNA or a truncated protein. Missense mutations are also not uncommon and usually cause disordered post-translational biosynthesis, like dimerization and multimerization defects. In general, these are mutations limited to individual families that occur either in the homozygous form or compound heterozygous form in accordance with the recessive mode of inheritance. There are no specific domains for mutations of type 3 VWD, since the above mutations can theoretically occur in the entire gene (☞ Figure 3.7).

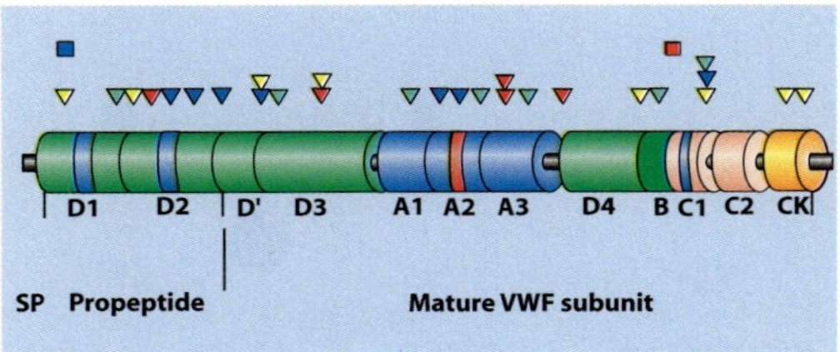


***Figure 3.7:*** Localization of mutations of severe type 3 von Willebrand disease. Blue triangles = small deletions; blue square = major deletion; red triangles = small insertions, red square = duplication, green triangles = nonsense mutations; yellow triangles = missense mutations; purple triangles = splice mutations.

Nevertheless, a mutation occurs very frequently in the countries around the Baltic Sea because of a founder effect. This is a one-base deletion in exon 18 (2435delC), which is found in half the chromosomes of Swedish patients with type 3 VWD, 20% of chromosomes of German patients, 20% of chromosomes of patients from Hungary and as many as 75% of chromosomes of Polish patients, but not in other patients analyzed to date, e.g. from the Netherlands or Turkey and only in one case in a compound heterozygous patients from Italy. Haplotype analyses showed that this is an "old" mutation that occurs in the different countries around the Baltic and probably has a common genetic origin (☞ Figure 3.8).

Patients with type 1 VWD often have VWF parameters that are also found in heterozygous trait carriers of type 3 VWD. However, the hypothesis that VWD type 1 might be due to a heterozygous type 3 defect has not been confirmed in most cases. The fact that relatives of type 3 patients often also complain of symptoms of bleeding may be a result of increased vigilance for bleeding symptoms and aggravation. Until recently, a systematic search for type 3 defects in patients with type 1 VWD was not carried out. It was not until a European study and a Canadian study on type 1 VWD that many, mostly new, mutations were identified. This study showed a new cluster of mutations, principally in the region of the D4 to the CK domain, that is, in the carboxyterminal part of VWF. These results confirm that type 1 VWD is an independent type. On the other hand, however, many of the study patients (32%) initially diagnosed as having type 1 VWD were classified as having the type 2 form.

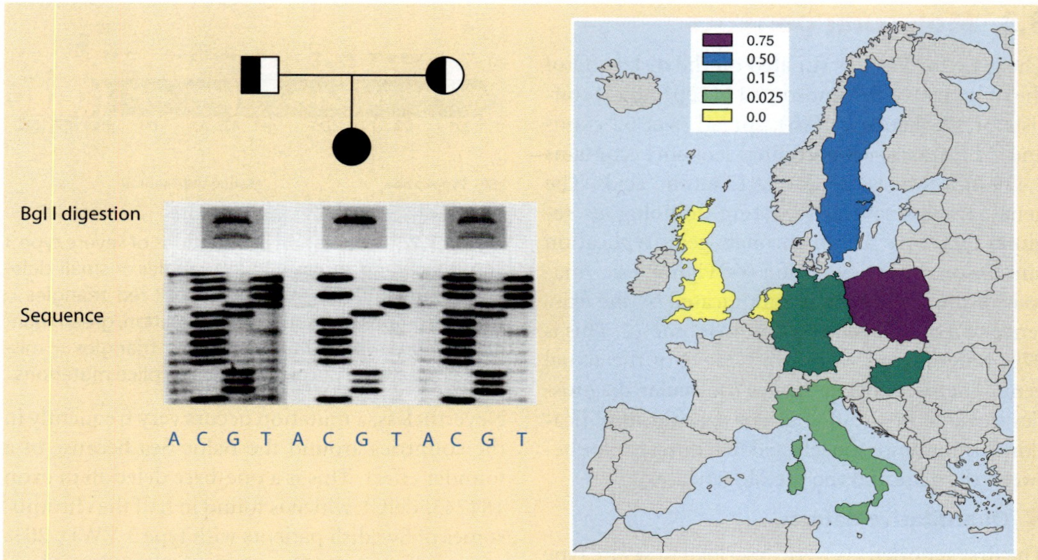


***Figure 3.8:*** Type 3 von Willebrand disease: Allele frequency of the most common mutation 2435delC in Europe. The concentration in the countries around the Baltic Sea suggests an old Baltic/Slavic mutation. Simple identification of the mutation by Bgl I restriction digestion in a family with type 3 VWD.

## Qualitative defects

The most interesting spectrum of mutations is shown by type 2 VWD (☞ Figure 3.9). This type is responsible for most of the marked heterogeneity of the clinical picture. Clinically, forms are found with an isolated disturbance of primary hemostasis, as in some subgroups of subtype 2A and some with isolated disturbance of secondary hemostasis as in subtype 2N. In most cases, the mode of inheritance is dominant, but the type 2N form shows recessive inheritance. To date, mutations in the VWF propeptide (phenotype IIC) have also been demonstrated to have, in general, recessive inheritance. The ongoing problems of classification of VWD are mainly a result of the heterogeneity of the type 2 (☞ Chapt. 4.).

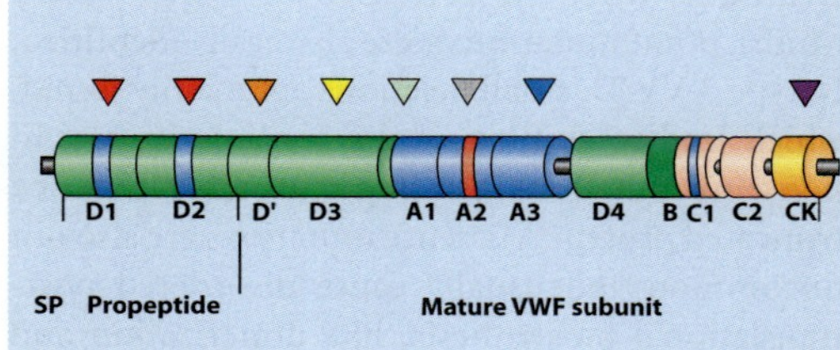


***Figure 3.9:*** Localization of the mutation clusters of type 2 von Willebrand disease. Red = mutations of VWD subtype 2A, subgroup IIC (multimerization defects), orange = mutations of VWD subtype 2N (FVIII binding defect), yellow = mutations of VWD subtype 2A, subgroup IIE/IIF (multimerization defects), green = mutations of VWD subtype 2B (increased affinity for GP Ib), gray = mutations of VWD subtype 2A subgroup IIA (with increased proteolysis), blue = collagen binding defects, purple = mutations of VWD subtype 2A, subgroup IID (dimerization defects).

Four different pathophysiological mechanisms are mainly responsible for type 2:

### 1. Pure functional disorders

The mutations identified so far affect either specific partial functions of VWF, e.g. the increased GP Ib binding in type 2B through mutations in the A1 domain, defective FVIII binding in type 2N in the FVIII binding region of the D' domain or isolated disturbance of collagen binding through mutations in the A3 domain.

▶ 2. Disorders of posttranslational biosynthesis, such as dimerization and multimerization with absence of large multimers

Mutations in the CK domain at the carboxy-terminal end of the VWF monomer (usually cysteine mutations) prevent effective dimerization. Since multimerization at the aminoterminal end is independent of prior dimerization at the carboxy-terminal end, dimers can nevertheless be formed, albeit via binding to the aminoterminal end. However, further multimerization is not then possible. Patients with homozygous mutations are phenotypically usually diagnosed as having type 3. heterozygous mutations are responsible for a special subgroup of type A, subgroup IID, which was termed type IID in the previous nomenclature (☞ Chapt. 4.).

Mutations in the D3 domain, the multimerization region of VWF containing many cysteines, impair the multimerization of dimers at the amino-terminal end and are responsible for subgroups IIE and IIF of type 2A. Patients with homozygous mutations may be diagnosed as having type 3 VWD. In heterozygous patients, large multimers may be absent or relatively reduced.

Mutations in the D1 and D2 domains of the VWF propeptide may also impair multimerization in the D3 domain. This is due to a decrease in the enzyme activity of the propeptide responsible for the linking of disulfide bonds. The phenotype (group IIC) with absence of large multimers is also classified as type 2A. However, unlike the other subgroups of type 2A, the inheritance is recessive. In contrast, a special form of subgroup IIC, phenotype IIC Miami, with mutations in the D3 domain, shows dominant inheritance. It differs from the normal phenotype IIC in that the VWF:Ag is raised.

▶ 3. Reduced resistance to the specific VWD-cleaving protease, ADAMTS13, resulting in increased breakdown of the large VWF multimers

Mutations in the A2 domain, which harbours the specific proteolytic site of cleavage between tyrosine 1605 and methionine 1606, lead to increased sensitivity to VWF-cleaving protease ADAMTS13. The result is a loss of the large multimers. The specific phenotype was previously called type IIA, which is now considered a subgroup of type 2A.

▶ 4. Impaired intracellular transport of the large VWD multimers

Other mutations in the A2 domain as well as in other regions of VWF lead to reduced secretion of the large VWF multimers and thus to a similar phenotype as the former type IIA. There are other mutations in the VWF propeptide that impair intracellular transport.

The possibility that exists today to ascribe specific mutations to specific VWD phenotypes may be used above all to improve the classification.

## 3.4. Role in hemostasis

### 3.4.1. Primary hemostasis

Flowing blood always shows a flow profile (☞ Figure 3.10). In this flow profile, the blood cells do not swim around in a disorganized manner but there is a clear distribution, with the large cells in the middle of the vessel lumen while the platelets, being smaller particles, are pushed out to the periphery of the stream. This is very important for hemostasis, as they have to interact with the injured vessel wall in order to be able to initiate primary hemostasis. Thus, anemia is always accompanied by a disorder of primary hemostasis, even though all other components of the system are completely intact.

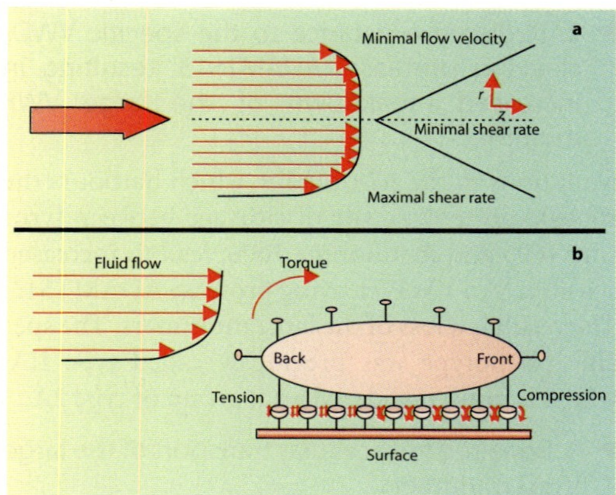


***Figure 3.10:*** **a:** The bloodstream in a cylindrical blood vessel may be considered as a series of layers, with the flow rate decreasing from the middle toward the periphery (arrows) at a lesser speed the further from the middle (arrows), with the velocity profile deviating somewhat from the parabolic profile since blood is not a pure fluid but a cell/fluid mixture. The shear forces change depending on the distance from the vessel wall. The lowest velocities and highest shearing rates are found immediately at the wall. Conversely, the velocity is greatest and the shear forces are lowest in the middle of the vessel.
**b:** Schematic representation of adhesion and how it is influenced by the prevailing shear forces. Adherent cells surrounded by a fluid are subject to tractive/rotatory forces that force the cells to roll. This movement arises through the spherical shape of the cell and the multiple binding sites on the vessel wall. The points of binding on the anterior side are compressed while on the opposite side a tractive force prevails, which results in release of the binding and to a rolling movement. Based on Ruggeri 2001, with permission.

VWF is found in an inactive form in the plasma, in the subendothelium, where it does not need to be activated since it is present in an active configuration, and in special storage organelles of the endothelial cells (Weibel-Palade bodies) and platelets (α-granules) from which it is released locally by appropriate stimuli. If there is bleeding in an area of flow with a higher shear rate than is present in veins, activated clotting factors are washed away before a normal clotting process might arise. Here, a matrix of platelets and VWF initially needs to form on which the consolidating clotting process can proceed. At the site of injury, there is first adhesion of platelets as a result of an interaction between the GP Ib on the platelet membrane, which does not require activation, and the VWF activated by shear stress. However, this is a reversible process, which does not result in firmly adherent platelets but only to a slowing in movement. It is worth noting that the adhesion takes place through threadlike outpouchings (tethers) of the platelets (☞ Figure 3.11).

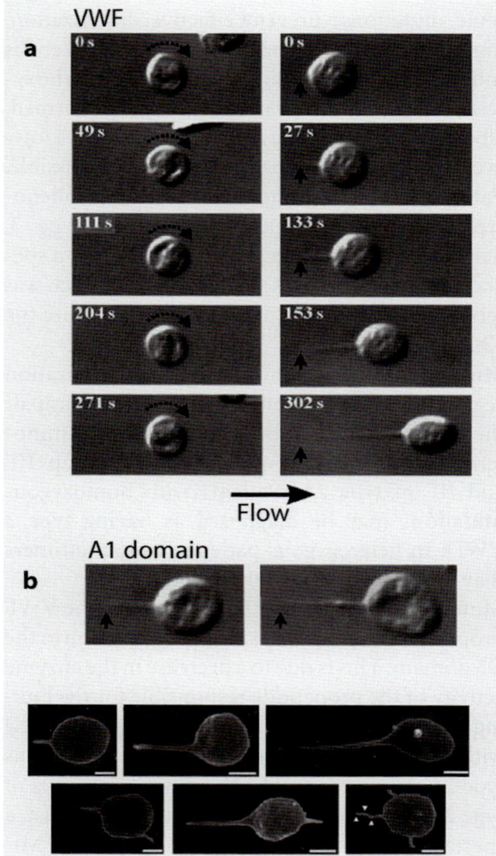


***Figure 3.11:*** **a:** Video image: If washed platelets are perfused over immobilized von Willebrand factor, they can either move without hindrance on the surface (left side) or they try to adhere firmly to the surface using fine tethers of the plasma membrane (right side), The small arrows show the points of adhesion that do not move during the period of observation. The formation of the tethers occurs both on the intact molecule as well as on the isolated A1 domain.
**b:** Electron microscopy views under the same conditions. From Dopheide et al. 2002, with permission.

As illustrated in Figure 3.12, the adhesion through tethers of the platelet membrane is advantageous in terms of energy compared with punctate adhesion, since these tethers are able to exert a much stronger force against the flow than punctate sites of contact.

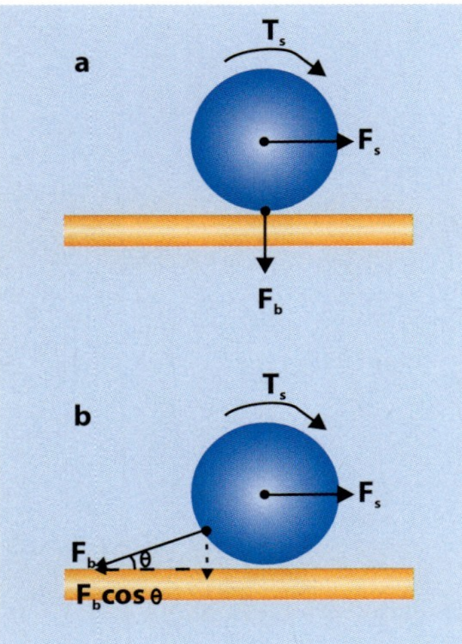


***Figure 3.12:*** Model showing the forces that are exerted on an adhering cell.
**a:** The adhering cell lying in a flow of fluid is subject to hydrodynamic shearing forces (Fs), which exert a rotatory moment (Ts) over the midpoint of the cell. The force (Fb) at the point of adhesion must counteract this rotatory moment. Binding with an intrinsic rapid rate of dissociation such as binding between VWF and GP Ib/IX has few possibilities for counteracting the rotatory moment under these conditions, resulting in translocation of the cell in the direction of the flow of fluid.
**b:** The formation of elongated tethers has clear mechanical advantages for the stable adhesion of cells. The tethers increase the horizontal force Fb, which considerably counteracts the force Fs with the force depending on the angle Q and the length of the tethers. Based on Dopheide et al. 2001.

However, there is only a slowed movement and never stable adhesion to the site of injury, if the GP IIb/IIIa receptor is not activated. In congenital deficiency (Glanzmann Naegel thrombasthenia) or in the case of a nonfunctioning receptor (e.g. GP IIb/IIIa antagonists) there is neither stable adhesion nor subsequent formation of an aggregate (☞ Figure 3.13).

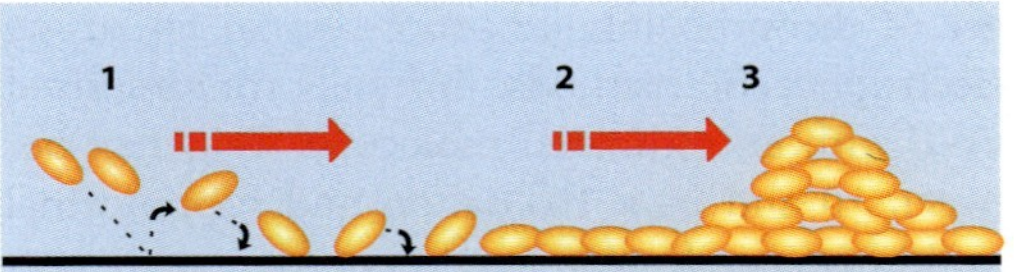


***Figure 3.13:*** Formation of a platelet thrombus: The formation of a platelet thrombus can be divided somewhat arbitrarily into three stages.
Stage **1**: Rolling. This involves transient adhesion, brought about by the immobilized VWF and the GP Ib/IX complex with platelets.
Stage **2**: Adhesion with simultaneous activation of platelets. The GP Ia/IIa and GP VI collagen receptors are dominant here.
Stage **3**: Consolidation of adhesion and aggregation: it is mediated by the GP IIb/IIIa platelet receptor and fibrinogen and/or VWF. Based on Kunicki 2001.

If the receptor is intact, platelet aggregation follows the initial adhesion through platelet-platelet interaction via bond formation between the GP IIb/IIIa receptor and fibrinogen, but also VWF. The mechanism described above is very important in regions with high shear forces but also plays a role in regions of low flow in veins and venules. The GP IIb/IIIa receptor is a receptor both for fibrinogen and VWF and thrombospondin. However, as fibrinogen is present in much higher quantities, the receptor is usually only occupied by fibrinogen. In afibrinogenemia (absence of fibrinogen in plasma and platelets), however, the receptor is free for VWF and by binding to this, VWF can stabilize hemostasis so that only a mild disturbance of hemostasis occurs. Approximately 4% of patients with this rare disease even have venous thromboembolism.

Primary hemostasis can function only if VWF is fully multimerized, since although in the absence of large multimers binding to a receptor can occur without hindrance, the formation of bonds cannot take place. In the presence of large amounts of defective VWF, there is therefore receptor blockade that is difficult to influence therapeutically. The local formation of supranormal multimers on the subendothelium induced by shearing forces as well as in the fluid phase has recently been described. These are very large molecules of more than 800 x $10^6$ dalton. These giant molecules can withstand considerable forces to initiate local primary hemostasis but require effective regulation by ADAMTS13 protease, otherwise there is the danger of thromboembolic processes. So far, using electrophoretic methods, normally multimerized vWF with an estimated molecular weight of between 10 and 20 x $10^6$ dalton and supranormal multimers (molecular weight approximately 40 x $10^6$ dalton) have been found. Recent investigations have shown, however, that special electron microscopic methods and measurements in laser light using different angles (light scattering) are needed in order to show the true size of this molecule, which may be in the region of several millimeters, which is a gigantic size for a protein. Thus, Moake et al. were able to visualize using an electron microscope elongated molecules with adhering platelets that were secreted by stimulated endothelium and reached a length of a few millimeters. Shankaran et al. proved the association between smaller molecules from the plasma and giant molecules of more than 800 x $10^6$ dalton using light diffraction of laser beams. They also showed that the quantities of detergence used for electrophoretic methods can break up these molecules into much smaller units.

### 3.4.2. Secondary hemostasis

In the D' domain, VWF has a binding region for FVIII (☞ Figure 3.6). There is an equilibrium between free VIII and VWF-bound FVIII. Approximately 95% of circulating FVIII is always bound to VWF. This corresponds to a FVIII level of only 0.01-0.05 U/mL in patients with type 3 VWD. Although every monomer of a VWF multimer can bind to a FVIII molecule, only about 2% of these binding sites are occupied by FVIII in vivo. VWF-bound FVIII is protected from proteolytic degradation. Without VWF, FVIII only has a half-life of 3 hours. Bound FVIII has a much longer half-life of 12-14 hours. As soon as the VWF concentration is no longer sufficient to stabilize FVIII effectively (approximately 0.3 U/mL), there is a reduction in FVIII both in type 1 and type 2. VWD 2N is a special type. Here, VWF has no FVIII binding capacity whatsoever, or it is greatly reduced. It results in a hemorrhagic diathesis similar to hemophilia A. Unlike the usual types of VWD, it involves a disturbance of secondary hemostasis.

# Classification and Pathogenesis

# 4. Classification and Pathogenesis

## 4.1. Introduction

The primary clinical feature for differentiating between the different types of von Willebrand disease (VWD) is the severity of the symptoms of bleeding. Mucosal bleeding and a tendency to hematomas are characteristic. Bleeding into joints and muscles, the main symptom of hemophilia, is rare and is found only in severe type 3 VWD, caused by the complete absence of von Willebrand factor (VWF) and very low FVIII levels, as well as in type 2N VWD in patients with isolated FVIII deficiency. Thus, simply by describing the spectrum of symptoms of bleeding in a patient can differentiate between a defect of primary hemostasis and a defect of secondary hemostasis or a combination of the two (☞ Table. 4.1).

| Type | 1 + 3 | 2A/2B/2M | 2N |
|---|---|---|---|
| Primary hemostasis | + | + | - |
| Secondary hemostasis | + | -/+ | + |

***Table 4.1:*** Classification of VWD according to phenotype. While the purely quantitatively defined types 1 and 3 show a similar reduction in the quantitative and functional parameters and thus primary and secondary hemostasis may be affected to the same extent, in the predominantly functional defects in subtypes 2A, 2B and 2M there is more an isolated impairment of primary hemostasis and in type 2N, because of the isolated FVIII reduction, only a marked disturbance of secondary hemostasis.

The main classification of VWD into 3 types has remained unchanged for years. However, with improved diagnostic techniques, the division into the different subtypes has changed. Thus, we diagnosed type 1, which previously was cited as representing 80-90%, in only 58% of patients. We found type 2, accounting for 40% of cases, to be much more common than previously thought (☞ Figure 4.1).

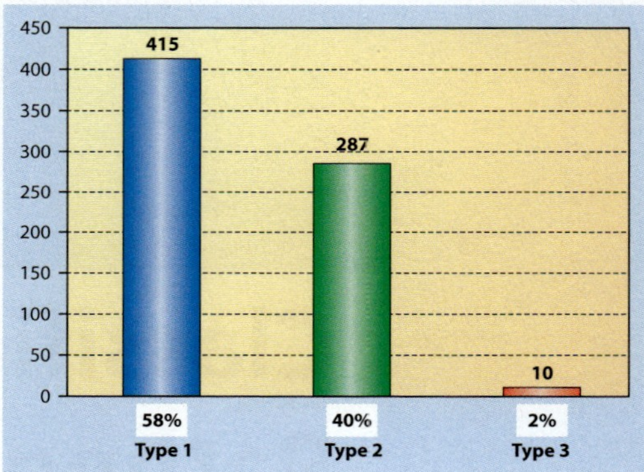


***Figure 4.1:*** Distribution of VWD types as a percentage (notifications from 2005).

The differentiation between type 1 with a reduced VWF concentration, and type 3, with complete VWF deficiency, as well as type 2, with qualitative defects regardless of the amount of VWF, is generally accepted. All attempts at subclassification nevertheless remain unsatisfactory because of lack of information about the biochemical and molecular basis of different variants or even more frequent types and subtypes of VWD. The first comprehensive classification into different types and subtypes of VWD was published by Ruggeri in 1987. Although this was more a list of all known variants of VWD integrated into a specific structure, it has nevertheless become the basis for the purposes of practical classification (☞ Table 4.2).

| Old | New |
|---|---|
| Type I | Type 1 |
| Types IIA, IIC, IID, IIE, IIF | Type 2A |
| Type I New York/Malmö, type IIB | Type 2B |
| Type B, type I Vicenza | Type 2M |
| - | Type 2N |
| Type III | Type 3 |

***Table 4.2:*** Von Willebrand disease - nomenclature.

Most of the subtypes were described on the basis of differences in multimer analysis (☞ Figure 4.2). In addition to quantitative and functional parameters, multimer analysis is still the method of choice for describing specific known or new subtypes of VWD.

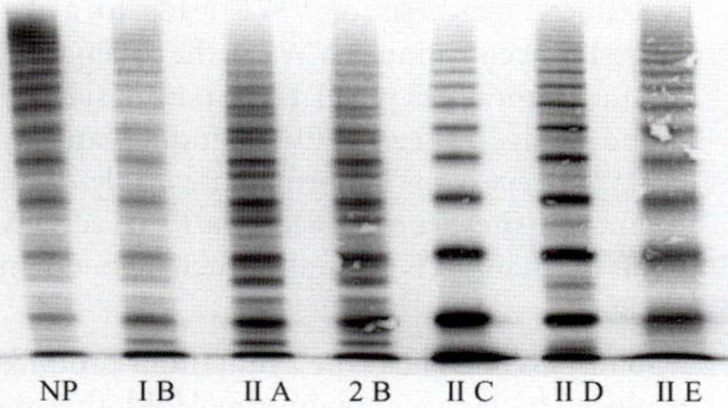


***Figure 4.2:*** Multimeric analysis of VWF of patients with different subtypes and subgroups of VWD compared with normal plasma in a medium resolution gel. The running direction is from top to bottom (i.e. the large multimers are in the upper part). In normal plasma and in plasma of subtypes IB, IIA and 2B, each oligomer consists of a triplet with a central band and an upper and lower subband. The remaining (sub)types show an abnormal band pattern. Roman numerals indicate the subgroups of subtype 2A.

One of the shortcomings of this initial classification was the fact that it was restricted to phenotype data given the lack of knowledge about the underlying mechanisms. On the other hand, the large number of different subtypes in this classification, although ideal for further biochemical and subsequent molecular investigations, was too complex for the practicing physician working with VWD patients. Additionally, functional von Willebrand factor defects that did not correlate with an abnormal multimeric structure were identified. This meant the definition of a qualitative defect had to be expanded. These issues were addressed by Sadler and Ginsburg in a revised classification of VWD. In this now valid classification, in addition to VWD 1 and VWD 3 as quantitative defects, VWD 2 is divided into 4 subgroups, among which VWD 2A covers variants with reduced platelet-dependent function based on loss of the large VWF multimers (high molecular weight multimers = HMWM) which are functionally most active in primary hemostasis. Variants with increased affinity for glycoprotein Ib (GP Ib) are termed type 2B VWD and encompass phenotypes with loss of large multimers but also those with a normal multimeric pattern. VWD 2M is based on platelet-dependent functional defects of VWF despite the presence of HMWM. VWD patients with defective FVIII binding of their VWF are diagnosed as VWD 2N (☞ Table 4.2).

We were able to classify most patients with type 2 VWD as subtype 2A (with loss of large multimers) using this classification (☞ Figure 4.3).

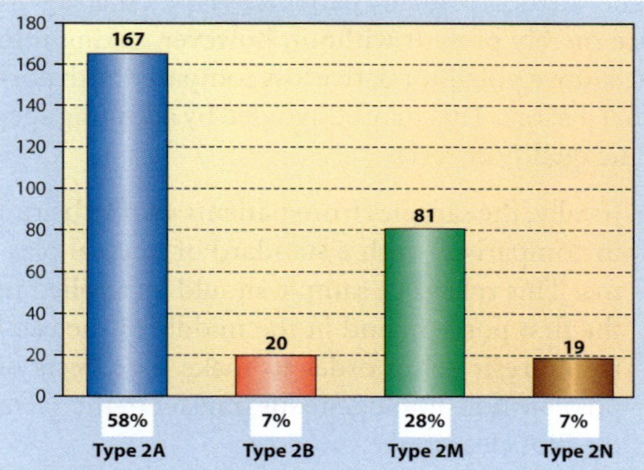


***Figure 4.3:*** Percentage distribution of the different type 2 VWD subtypes (results from 2005).

## 4.2. Critical appraisal of the current classification

An ideal classification should be equally useful to the clinician, geneticist and molecular biologist. This was not the case for the initial new classification. Since clinical work is patient-oriented, a practical classification is the top priority for the clinician. However, increasing knowledge about the pathophysiological mechanisms of VWF mutations and their importance for the structure and function of VWF as well as their correlation with a specific clinical phenotype has enabled a differential classification of VWD. The types and subtypes of VWD should ideally be defined through a clear correlation between phenotype and genotype. The initial new classification, however, was based mainly on a description of phenotype. A revised version of the current classification was adopted at the last working meeting of the Scientific and Standardization Committee (SSC) of the International Society of Thrombosis and Hemostasis (ISTH) in Oslo in June 2006. Some of the criticisms were addressed in the new version.

### 4.2.1. Type 1 VWD (VWD 1)

In VWD 1, all VWF parameters are equally reduced and the VWF multimers cannot be distinguished qualitatively from those in normal plasma. In clinical practice, however, the lack of standardization of multimer analysis has led to difficulties in differentiating between a real or artifactual loss of HMWM. This is principally due to insufficient transfer of HMWM during the Western blotting process. It appears to be common practice in many laboratories to qualify patients as type 1 if HMWM are merely present without, however, taking into account a possible relative loss compared with normal plasma. This may be avoided by adopting specific quality criteria:

- Ideally, the samples from patients should be run in comparison with a standard of normal plasma. This reference sample should be applied in the first position and in the middle of the electrophoresis gel in order to make the effects of possible non-homogeneous transfer of the gel to the blot clear to see.
- HMWM should be present and should appear with increased intensity compared with the smaller multimers.
- Individual triplets in the low-molecular-weight region should be separated from each other by a clear space.
- A reference sample from a normal platelet lysate is needed to demonstrate particularly large, so-called supranormal multimers for comparison. This is best done by using a medium-resolution gel (e.g. 1.5% agarose). Gels with a higher resolution are needed to more accurately show the triplet structure of individual multimers. However, even under physiological conditions, in addition to the concentration of VWF, the amount of high-molecular-weight multimers may also markedly differ because of, for example, stimulated secretion of VWF and thereby have an effect on abnormal distribution of the different large multimers. In the worst instance, this may erroneously suggest a normal result.

In the past, it was very difficult to tackle these problems, with the tests being repeated several times, producing contradictory results. Today, however, the correlation of specific phenotypes with specific molecular defects can aid in defining these subtypes and thus provide a clear basis for a clear diagnosis.

#### 4.2.1.1. Pathogenesis

Three mechanisms are known to be able to give rise to type 1 VWD:

1. Reduced synthesis of VWF leads to a decreased concentration of VWF in the plasma and not uncommonly in platelets too (site of synthesis and storage). Since the FVIII binding capacity of VWF is very high (in normal cases, only 2% of the binding sites are occupied), the FVIII activity in this mechanism is generally much higher than VWF:Ag.

2. Some heterozygous type 2 mutations produce products showing highly abnormal folds that are destroyed intracellularly and thus are not secreted. The normal dimers produced in lower concentrations remain; these undergo the normal process of multimerization, storage and secretion. The constellation FVIII:C >VWF:Ag is also typically found here.

3. Accelerated clearance in the circulation. In this case, the FVIII/VWF complex is removed from the plasma. Thus, FVIII:C and VWF:Ag are similarly reduced (ratio of FVIII:C to VWF:Ag around 1). The accelerated clearance in blood group 0 compared with other blood groups has long been known. The clearance is even more rapid in the Bombay phenotype. In type 1 VWD, blood group 0 is found in approximately 70% and is clearly overrepresented compared with the normal population and the other types of VWD. In the Vicenza subtype (where classification into type 1 or type 2 is currently controversial), the elimination from the plasma is accelerated in such a way that neither the supranormal multimers can be broken down nor can a normal triplet structure be formed. In the other patients with type 1, these changes cannot be detected using current methods.

### 4.2.2. Type 3 VWD (VWD 3)

The most severe form of type 3 VWD is easy to diagnose because of the complete deficiency of VWF and its functions. In most cases, major deletions and truncating mutations at a molecular level are found to be the cause of severe VWD 3. A few homozygous missense mutations have also been described. In some of these, low amounts of VWF can be detected but with an abnormal multimeric structure. The VWF antigen (VWF:Ag) is severely reduced. Clinically, patients with these mutations cannot be differentiated from other type 3 patients with truncating mutations. It thus appears advisable to continue to define these patients as also having type 3 although some of them are found to have residual concentrations of VWF using highly sensitive methods.

### 4.2.3. Type 2 VWD (VWD 2)

Subtyping of VWD 2 is the most difficult aspect in the classification of VWD. This is due to the enormous heterogeneity of the functional and structural defects. Among these, purely functional defects, such as impaired FVIII binding in VWD 2N, may be easily diagnosed and this phenotype may be designated as a subtype in its own right. However, other subtypes that have only a few features in common are grouped together as VWD 2A although the molecular mechanisms and also the inheritance may be very heterogeneous. The current classification is shown in comparison to the previous classification in Table 4.1.

#### 4.2.3.1. Pathogenesis

In principle, five different molecular pathophysiological mechanisms are responsible for type 2, which may be effective alone or in combination:

▶ 1. Purely functional disturbances

The mutations identified so far concern either specific partial functions of VWF, such as increased GP Ib binding in type 2B through mutations in the A1 domain, defective FVIII binding in type 2N in the FVIII binding region of the D' domain or the isolated defect of collagen binding as a result of mutations in the A3 domain. Mutations that lead to a pathological interaction with GP Ib, even if the large multimers are present, induce type 2M.

▶ 2. Disorders of post-translational biosynthesis, such as dimerization and multimerization with absence of large multimers

Mutations in the CK domain at the carboxyterminal end of the VWF monomer (usually cysteine mutations) prevent effective dimerization. Since multimerization at the aminoterminal end is independent of prior dimerization at the carboxyterminal end, dimers may nevertheless be formed but via binding to the aminoterminal end. Further multimerization is not, however, possible. Patients with compound heterozygous or homozygous mutations in this region are usually phenotypically diagnosed as type 3. Heterozygous mutations are responsible for a specific subgroup of type 2A, dimerization defects, which were termed type IID in the old nomenclature (☞ Chapt. 5.3.1.).
Mutations in the D3 domain, the multimerization region of VWF rich in cysteine, reduce the multimerization of dimers at the aminoterminal end and cause subgroup IIE of type 2A. Patients with homozygous mutations may be diagnosed as having VWD type 3. In heterozygous patients, the large multimers may either be absent or (more frequently) relatively reduced.
Mutations in the D1 and D2 domain of VWF propeptide may also impair multimerization in the D3 domain. This is due to reduced enzyme activity in the propeptide necessary for the formation of disulfide bonds. The IIC phenotype with absence of large multimers is also classed under type 2A, but, unlike the other subgroups of type 2A, the inheritance is recessive. However, a special form of subgroup IIC, phenotype IIC Miami, with mutations in the D3 domain, has dominant inheritance. It differs from the normal phenotype IIC in that there is increased VWF:Ag and a trace of proteolytic fragments. Classification of a particularly severe type 2A (subgroup IIE) is thus possible.

▶ 3. Reduced resistance to proteolysis by the VWF-cleaving protease ADAMTS13 resulting in increased breakdown of the large VWF multimers

Mutations in the A2 domain that flank the specific proteolytic cleavage site between tyrosine 1605 and methionine 1606 lead to increased sensitivity to the VWF cleaving protease ADAMTS 13. A consequence of this is loss of the large multimers. The previous designation for this phenotype was type IIA. Today, it is considered as a subgroup of type 2A.

▶ 4. Disturbed intracellular transport of the large VWF multimers

Other mutations in the A2 domain as well as in other regions of VWF lead to reduced secretion of the large VWF multimers and thus to a similar phenotype to the previous type IIA. Other mutations that impair intracellular transport occur in the VWF propeptide.

▶ 5. Increased breakdown of VWF in the circulation

Cysteine mutations in the D3 domain and mutation R1205H lead to rapid clearance of VWF, the mechanism for which is still poorly understood.

▶ 6. Abnormal folding of the molecule, which does not prevent storage and secretion but results in VWF with decreased reactivity (type 2M)

The VWF from patients with type 2M cannot react or reacts to only a slight degree as a result of abnormal folding of the molecule. As a result of this, supranormal multimers are often not processed and the formation of a triplet structure cannot proceed. The VWF:FVIIIB to VWF:Ag ratio is usually not reduced; some patients with a combination of 2M/2N are, however, described.

The molecular mechanisms are very diverse but show a very good correlation between phenotype and genotype. Thus, most subtypes of VWD type 2 can be attributed to specific mutations in defined domains of VWF (☞ Figure 5.9). This possibility of attributing specific mutations to specific VWD phenotypes may be used above all to improve the classification.

### 4.2.3.2. Type 2A VWD

VWD 2A includes all patients with absence of, or a reduction in, high-molecular-weight multimers. At the same time, there is a reduction in platelet-dependent function. This type includes subtypes Ib, 1-platelet-discordant, IIA, IIA-1, IIA-2, IIA-3, IIC, IIE, IIF, IIG, IIH and II-I (☞ Figure 4.4).

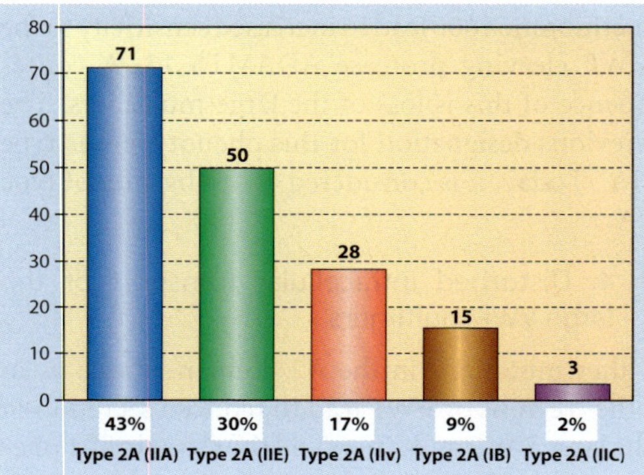


***Figure 4.4:*** Percentage distribution of the most common subgroups of subtype 2A VWD (notifications from 2005). IIv = abnormal "smeary" triplet structure (subgroup that has not so far been defined).

The mechanisms that result in a reduction in, or absence of, large multimers are nevertheless very different and the pattern of inheritance of these subtypes also varies. The reduction in HMWM in type 2A is explained either on the basis of disordered intracellular transport (group 1 mutations) or increased proteolysis of these through the VWF specific protease (group 2 mutations). The first mutations were published in 1989. The different mutations that lead to this type are localized in the A2 domain of VWF, or affect cysteine 1272 or cysteine 1458 in the A1 domain. Most of these mutations are listed in the VWF mutation database (http://www.VWF.group.shef.ac.uk/). A further reason for deficiency of the large multimers is defective posttranslational modification. Included in this are defects of dimerization at the carboxy-terminal end of VWF, as in subtype IID, and defects of further polymerization of VWF dimers to multimers at the amino terminus. The latter multimerization defects may be caused by mutations in the D1 and D2 domain of the VWF propeptide. These domains are necessary to catalyze the intermolecular disulfide bond formation in the D3 domain of mature VWF. As may be expected, mutations in the D3 domain themselves may cause multimerization defects. These are essentially cysteine mutations. While mutations in the D1 and D2 domain are correlated with VWD subtype IIC, mutations in the D3 domain are found in VWD subtype IIE and VWD IIF as well as in subtype IIC Miami. Most subtypes of VWD 2A are dominantly inherited, apart from subtype IIC, which has recessive inheritance. In addition to a reduction in, or loss of, large multimers, the multimeric pattern in subtypes IIE and IIF shows an abnormal triplet structure with absence of the external subbands but with a prominent inner band of the triplet. In low-resolution gels, the central band appears wider. A similar phenotype was also originally described as VWD type IIH. Although being similar in terms of the multimeric pattern of the VWF from plasma, patients with subtypes IIE and IIF differ from each other in relation to the multimeric pattern of platelet VWF. Whereas in subtype IIE, the defect is found in the plasma and platelets, the typical multimeric pattern in type IIF is only restricted to the plasma. Surprisingly, the IIE/IIF phenotype is very frequent and accounts for approximately 30% of all patients with type 2A VWD. In these patients, we have identified a cluster of mutations in the VWF D3 domain (☞ Figure 5.9), which principally affect cysteine residues, which in turn participate directly or indirectly in intermolecular disulfide bond formation at the amino terminus of the mature VWF, the essential domain for VWF multimerization. The multimerization defect may be reproduced through recombinant expression of mutant VWF.

#### 4.2.3.3. Type 2B VWD (VWD 2B)

A further reason for the absence of large multimers is the increased affinity of VWF for platelet glycoprotein Ib (GP Ib) in patients with VWD 2B. In some of these patients, the multimers are nevertheless normal as in VWD 2B New York/Malmö. The mode of inheritance is dominant. Type 2B may be well defined through the test of ristocetin-induced platelet agglutination and through localization of the accompanying mutations in a limited region of the A1 domain. The first candidate mutations were reported in 1991. Numerous other mutations are listed in the VWF mutation database (http://www.shef.ac.uk/VWF/mutations.html).

#### 4.2.3.4. Type 2M VWD (VWD 2M)

This type, which also has dominant inheritance, includes patients with reduced platelet-dependent function of VWF that is not due to absence of HMWM. No account is taken of other differentiating properties, such as an abnormal structure of individual multimers or the presence of particularly large, so-called supranormal multimers, as in VWD type 2M Vicenza. Most mutations that have been described so far are concentrated in the A1 domain of VWF. The subtype VWD 2M Vicenza is associated with a specific mutation (R1205H) in the D3 domain of VWF in most families. The diagnostic problem in VWD 2M is similar to the situation in VWD 1, since the quality of multimer analysis leaves room for interpretation. Indeed, it was found that mutations in the A1 domain in patients previously classified as having VWD 1 were correlated with a relative reduction in large multimers on re-examination, suggesting the correct diagnosis to be more VWD 2A. Thus, careful reevaluation of patients with VWD 2M and patients with VWD 1 appears to be necessary, especially in cases where there is a discrepancy between VWF:Ag and ristocetin cofactor VWF:RCo or VWF:CB. In nearly all patients with type 2M, we find an abnormal multimeric pattern. Proteolytic subbands (triplets) are clearly reduced or completely absent indicating reduced proteolysis. Instead, amorphous material lying around the central bands is seen, which also occupies the usually "VWF-free" space between the individual oligomers. In addition, the migration speed of the oligomers is not uncommonly increased and, because of the lack of adhesive function, supranormal multimers persist, indicating defective cleavage by ADAMTS13 (☞ Figure 4.5).

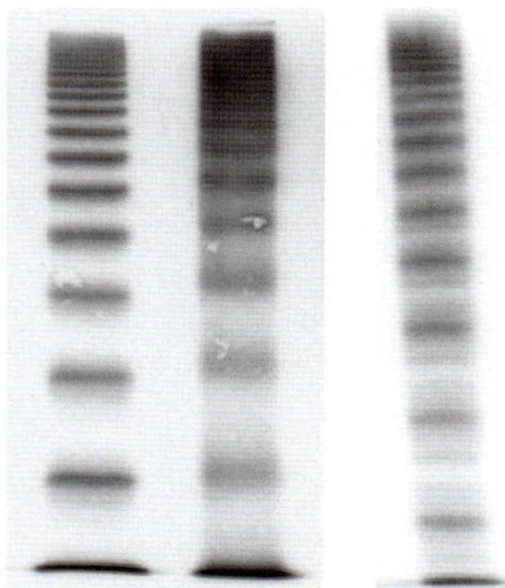


***Figure 4.5:*** Multimeric analysis of VWF from patients with type 2A (subtype IIE) vs 2M (v) compared with normal plasma in a medium-resolution gel. The running direction is from top to bottom (i.e. the large multimers are in the upper part). In normal plasma, each oligomer is composed of a triplet with a central band and an upper and lower subband. In type IIE, the large multimers are present in much lower concentrations and the external subbands of the triplet are absent. In type 2M, the large multimers are even present in increased concentrations; a triplet structure is completely absent. Instead, the area around the central bands is filled with amorphous material. This makes the pattern appear smeary. NP = normal mixed plasma; (sm) stands for smeary. The right lane (NP) is from a separate gel.

#### 4.2.3.5. VWD type Normandy (VWD 2N)

This type encompasses patients with a defect in the FVIII binding region of VWF. Patients may either be homozygous or compound heterozygous for a FVIII binding defect, or compound heterozygous for a FVIII binding defect and a null allele. Accordingly, the phenotype may either mistakenly suggest hemophilia A or may additionally be accompanied by a reduced VWF:Ag. Some mutations also alter the structure of VWF multimers. The mode of inheritance is recessive. This type is well defined by the FVIII binding defect and by mutations in the FVIII binding region (D' domain) or in direct proximity. Since all other parameters, including the concentration of VWF, may be normal, this type may only be differentiated from hemophilia A through the so-called FVIII binding assay (☞ Figure 5.7). In individual cases, the FVIII in these patients may also be in the region of 1% and thus in the range of severe hemophilia.

# Diagnosis

# 5. Diagnosis

## 5.1. Biochemical parameters

von Willebrand disease can be detected in about 1% of the population using laboratory tests (1-3). However, only a small number of these individuals have definite symptoms (1:3,000 to 1:10,000). A prevalence of 125 cases per million of the population has been estimated for Sweden, a country with a homogeneous population and very good records for patients with a bleeding diathesis. Whether for the remainder it is a purely laboratory phenomenon or a clinically relevant disease can only be determined through clinical observation.

An additional complication is the fact that circulating von Willebrand factor depends on the blood group. VWF in individuals with blood group 0 has a much shorter half-life in the blood than in individuals with other blood groups. As a result, the concentration is on average 0.25 U/mL lower. Thus, for blood group 0, a VWF concentration of 0.35 U/mL is still normal, while it is clearly reduced for the other blood groups. VWF does not have an association with sex. It does, however, increase from the age of 40 onwards by about 0.06 U/mL for each decade. In addition, VWF reacts like an acute phase protein. This means that it may be increased short term (stress) or long term (pregnancy, malignant disease). Thus, a personal and family history is essential for classification in patients with von Willebrand disease or normal individuals with a low VWF. The normal VWF concentration of 0.4 to 1.6 U/mL is suboptimal. Thus, the adhesiveness of platelets, for example, increases up to a concentration of 3 U/mL. At 0.4 U/mL, a critical limit is reached. VWF is still able to cope with normal demands even under conditions of stress such as injuries or surgical operations, but each further disturbance of hemostasis (e.g. ASS use, infections) can no longer be compensated and leads to possibly dangerous hemorrhage.

Platelet VWF is released locally by thrombin. This greatly increases the local VWF concentration in injured vascular areas and can also compensate for low plasma VWF levels. Thus, for the same plasma VWF concentration, the bleeding tendency in patients with reduced platelet VWF is much greater than in patients with normal intraplatelet VWF. Unfortunately, there is not yet a standard for platelet VWF and nor are there methods established for the necessary lysis of platelets or a reference (U/$10^{11}$ platelets, U/mg protein, % of a platelet pool). There is therefore no recognized lower limit for platelet VWF.

In fact, differentiating between patients with mild von Willebrand disease and normal individuals with a low VWF concentration is very important. On the one hand, normal individuals may be classed as "bleeders" throughout their lives (emergency or hemophiliac card), while on the other, patients who, because of an increase in VWF short term have normal parameters, are wrongly classified as normal. Several investigations are consequently often necessary in order to confirm or discard a suspected diagnosis. Because of usually raised and very variable VWF parameters in neonates and early infancy, reliable levels can only be obtained from the 6$^{th}$ month of life onward, except in patients with severe type 3 VWD and some patients with type 2 disease. However, mild forms cannot be reliably diagnosed until after this period.

### 5.1.1. Investigation procedure

In the identification of a disorder of hemostasis, a detailed history is very important and directs subsequent laboratory diagnostic tests. Evidence from the history of a disorder of hemostasis will suggest special investigations even if the global clotting tests are normal because of a lack of sensitivity.

The marked heterogeneity of VWF defects mirrors the heterogenous bleeding symptoms in patients with different types. In patients who have sufficient VWF:Ag to stabilize FVIII in the plasma to such an extent that the FVIII activity exceeds 0.3 U/mL, primary hemostasis is predominantly affected. These are patients with type 1 disease and a mild course but also many patients with type 2 disease. In the remaining patients, both primary and secondary hemostasis are affected. Patients whose VWF does not stabilize FVIII (type 2N) show an atypical response. These patients lack the characteristic symptoms of a disorder of primary hemostasis. Depending on the residual activity of factor VIII, they behave like patients with mild, and more rarely, moderate hemophilia. The flowchart shown in Figure 5.1 is recommended for differentiating between a diagnosis of VWD and hemophilia.

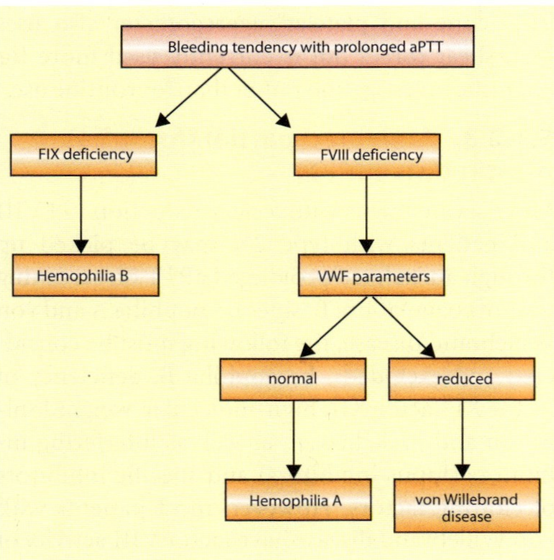


***Figure 5.1:*** Flow chart for differentiating between hemophilia and VWD.

## Symptoms of bleeding

(☞ Table 2.1)

The methods used to investigate suspected von Willebrand disease may be divided into screening diagnostic tests, extended diagnostic tests and special diagnostic tests (☞ Table 5.1).

| Screening diagnostic tests |
|---|
| • Bleeding time<br>• Filter method with high shear stress (e.g. PFA-100)<br>• Partial thromboplastin time (aPTT) |
| **Extended diagnostic tests** |
| • VWF antigen (VWF:Ag)<br>• Ristocetin cofactor activity (VWF:RCo)<br>• FVIII activity (FVIII:C) |
| **Special diagnostic tests** |
| • VWF collagen binding capacity (VWF:CB)<br>• Ristocetin-induced platelet aggregation (RIPA)<br>• Multimer analysis<br>• VWF parameters in platelets<br>• FVIII binding capacity of VWF (VWF:FVIIIB) |

***Table 5.1:*** Investigation procedure in the case of suspected von Willebrand disease (characteristic constellations of findings in types of von Willebrand disease are shown in Table 5.2).

## 5.1.2. Screening diagnostic tests

### 5.1.2.1. Bleeding time

The bleeding time is a global test of primary hemostasis. It reveals qualitative and quantitative platelet disorders, quantitative and qualitative defects of VWF, vessel wall disturbances and disturbances as a result of a reduction in the erythrocyte count. A prolonged bleeding time is characteristic and was also repeatedly described in the first publications. The prolongation of the bleeding time is, however, very variable in mild forms of von Willebrand dis-

| Type | Mode of inheritance | Bleeding time | FVIII:C | VWF:Ag | VWF:RCo | VWF:CB | RIPA | Multimers in plasma | Multimers in platelets |
|---|---|---|---|---|---|---|---|---|---|
| 1 | AD | ↑/n | ↓ | ↓ | ↓ | ↓ | n/↓ | All present | All present |
| 2A | AD/AR | ↑ | ↓/n | ↓ | ↓ | ↓ | ↓/n | Large and/or medium-sized absent | All present or like plasma |
| 2B | AD | ↑ | ↓/n | ↓/n | ↓ | ↓ | ↑↑ | Large absent | All present |
| 2M | AD | ↑ | ↓/n | ↓ | ↓/n | n/↓ | ↓/n | All present | All present |
| 2N | AR | n | ↓↓ | n/↓ | n/↓ | n/↓ | n | All present | All present |
| 3 | AR | ↑↑ | ↓↓ | nd | nd | nd | nd | nd | nd |

***Table 5.2:*** Characteristic constellation of findings in different types of von Willebrand disease.
n = normal; nd = not detectable; AD = autosomal dominant; AR = autosomal recessive.

ease and is often found to be normal. It is important to use a standardized method. In older children and adults, automatic blades for measurement of the bleeding time devised by Mielke have proved their worth, but this method has not been demonstrated to be superior to the less traumatic and cheaper method for measuring the bleeding time devised by Ivy. The Ivy method is the preferred method especially in small children. Often, the bleeding time must be determined several times precisely in mild cases of type 1 in order to measure a prolongation. Here, too, the bleeding time is not regarded as a sensitive test for von Willebrand disease. After infusion of FVIII/von Willebrand factor concentrates or DDAVP, the Duke bleeding time is preferred as a control parameter by some authors because it can be normalized more readily than the Ivy bleeding time. Whether in addition to its diagnostic importance, measurement of the bleeding time also has prognostic significance for the severity of bleeding is a subject of discussion.

The bleeding time is becoming increasingly less important as a result of the more sensitive in vitro bleeding time methods (☞ below), which are independent of the investigator and also atraumatic. It is no longer an essential method for the diagnosis of von Willebrand disease.

### 5.1.2.2. Filter methods with high shear stress

The in vitro bleeding time using the Thrombostat 4000 and its successor the PFA 100 and the O'Brien filter method measure the time until a specific capillary is sealed after the flow of blood through a specially coated filter. These methods work with a shear stress that is similar to the shear stress found in arterioles. Thus, the closure time is dependent on primary hemostasis alone. The closure time is influenced by VWF as well as the platelet count and platelet function and the hematocrit. These methods are much more sensitive in patients with mild von Willebrand disease than the in vivo bleeding time. However, even using these methods, differentiation is not always possible between normal individuals and patients with mild von Willebrand disease in the so-called gray area between 0.35 U/mL and 0.60 U/mL. The centrifugation method of Wenzel's working group involves much lower costs in terms of equipment and materials and also appears to yield comparable results. However, more experience needs to be gained for a conclusive assessment.

The "cone and platelet" aggregometer also uses high shear forces but is currently used more for scientific investigation rather than for routine use.

### 5.1.2.3. Activated partial thromboplastin time (aPTT)

More severe forms with a clear reduction in FVIII and patients with type 2N may be picked up through an isolated prolonged aPTT on screening tests of coagulation. Besides hemophilia A and von Willebrand disease, the following must be considered and excluded: hemophilia B, deficiency of factor XI, factor XII, high-molecular-weight kininogen and prekallikrein as well as interfering inhibitors (lupus inhibitors) and specific inhibitors of clotting factors. However, most patients with von Willebrand disease have factor VIII activity of more than 0.3 U/mL and thus are not detected by a prolonged aPTT. Mild FXII reductions are relatively frequent and the aPTT reacts even with small decreases in FXII activity. Thus, some patients are picked up during diagnostic assessment of a prolonged aPTT. Combined FXII and VWF deficiency was previously classified as a special type (von Willebrand disease San Diego). However, it was recently shown that this association is purely coincidental.

The aPTT is now almost exclusively determined using automated or semi-automated devices. There is thus no longer the previous variation because of the variable determination of the point of clotting. However, major differences in relation to the sensitivity for mild factor VIII decreases still exist because of the composition of the different commercial reagents. There are no comparison studies on the detection of mild forms of von Willebrand disease. However, as this test only detects a factor VIII decrease, comparison studies using plasma samples from patients with hemophilia A may be used. These studies have shown that the aPTT is not a sensitive test for subhemophilia because of the substantial biological, pathological and analytical variation and thus is also not suitable for von Willebrand disease.

#### 5.1.2.4. Adhesion/retention

VWF is the most important protein for normal platelet adhesion, especially in vascular regions with a high flow rate. Accordingly, quantitative and/or qualitative disorders of VWF are accompanied by reduced platelet adhesion. Besides measurement of the bleeding time, measurement of the ability of platelets to adhere is the only functional test for the activity of VWF. However, the current conventional Baumgartner or Sakriassen adhesion tests are not suitable for routine investigations. The Hellem or Salzman glass bead filter methods measure both the adhesion as well as the aggregation of platelets and are now used only rarely. The only truly practicable methods that determine the function of VWF under high shear stress are the in vitro bleeding time methods (☞ above), which will probably replace the bleeding time in the near future.

#### 5.1.2.5. Platelet count

Measurement of the platelet count is used more for the exclusion of another disorder of primary hemostasis than for the diagnosis of von Willebrand disease. In patients with type 2B and pseudo (platelet-type) von Willebrand disease, there is found to be consistent or intermittent thrombocytopenia, depending on the reactivity of the VWF, indicating increased interaction between the platelet receptor (GP Ib) and the A1 domain of VWF.

### 5.1.3. Extended diagnostic tests

#### 5.1.3.1. Assay of the FVIII/VWF complex

All tests used for assaying the FVIII/VWF complex need to use standards that have been calibrated to the WHO standard. Each laboratory is required to determine its own normal ranges. Whether separate normal ranges for patients with blood group 0 and non-0 are necessary is still a matter of controversy.

#### 5.1.3.2. Factor VIII (FVIII)

FVIII is only indirectly affected in von Willebrand disease, with the exception of type 2N. Provided sufficient VWF (>0.3 U/mL) is available to stabilize FVIII in plasma, patients with von Willebrand disease have normal factor VIII activity. The aPTT is thus also not a sensitive parameter. However, since FXII reductions in von Willebrand disease are not uncommon, von Willebrand disease may be picked up through a prolonged aPTT in routine testing even if FVIII activity is normal. For the 2N variant, assay of FVIII activity is an essential diagnostic test.

The activity of FVIII is usually determined in the aPTT system with specific deficient plasma. In recent years, assays using chromogenic substrates less subject to disturbance have gained in importance, but are not very suitable for individual assays because of the configuration of the assay kit. Commercial kits are marketed by many manufacturers of clotting reagents.

FVIII:Ag is assayed using immunoradiometric or enzymoimmunological methods with the help of human or monoclonal antibodies. Assay of FVIII:Ag is of little significance for diagnostic purposes.

#### 5.1.3.3. VWF Antigen (VWF:Ag)

Assay of VWF:Ag is indispensable for the diagnosis, since only through this can a distinction be made between reduced and dysfunctional VWF.

The VWF:Ag in platelets should be included in diagnostic testing for the reasons outlined above. However, the lack of standardization makes comparison with the results of other laboratories difficult.

The test previously used most often, the Laurell electroimmunoassay method modified by Zimmerman, is now by and large obsolete. The limit of detection of this method is between 0.05 and 0.1 U/mL. Moreover, the molecule size influences the speed of migration with the result that in type 2 too high concentrations are often measured. IRMA or ELISA methods, both using poly- or monoclonal antisera, are much more sensitive and have better reproducibility at low concentrations. The rapid latex-based methods that have only recently become available allow a relatively cheap, quick (about 15 minutes) and precise assay. Commercial kits from several companies are available for all described non-radioactive methods.

The VWF:Ag is reduced in more than 80% of patients with von Willebrand disease. In mild forms of von Willebrand disease, the lower range of normal may be reached, especially in situations of stress. The blood group relationship of the FVIII/VWF complex in the so-called gray area between

0.35 and 0.6 U/mL also results in difficulties. However, investigation of suspected von Willebrand disease is incomplete if the assay of the VWF concentration is not combined with a method that assesses the functional capability of VWF.

#### 5.1.3.4. Ristocetin cofactor activity (VWF:RCo)

In vitro, platelets react with each other in the presence of ristocetin and VWF. Using washed platelets, a property of VWF, the ristocetin cofactor activity, may be quantitatively determined.

Principle of the method: Normal platelets, a constant quantity of ristocetin and standard or patient plasma dilutions are made to react under suitable conditions and the activity of the plasma being tested is compared with that of standard plasma. Fresh and fixed, lyophilized or frozen platelets are suitable. However, fresh platelets can only keep for a short time. Preserved platelets are thus usually used. The reaction may take place in an aggregometer, on test plates or in a platelet counter. Ristocetin may be replaced by botrocetin. Commercial washed and fixed test platelets are currently provided by two manufacturers (Dade/Behring and Mölab). The Dade/Behring reagent was specially developed for macroscopic agglutination, while the Mölab reagent was developed for aggregometry. However, both reagents may be used for other methods. The VWF:RCo may be automatically assayed in the Dade/Behring coagulation analyzer. The great variability of the methods, which has been known since the very early days of tests for VWF:RCo, is problematic and despite much effort cannot be eliminated.

An ELISA method enabling better standardization was recently published. Binding of VWF is on immobilized recombinant GP Ib. A comparable sensitivity and specificity to that found in the assay of VWF:Ag is achieved. The test can replace the RIPA test (☞ below) by varying the ristocetin concentration. However, this test is not yet commercially available.

The ristocetin cofactor behaves like the VWF:Ag (☞ above). For patients with a mild form of von Willebrand disease, it is somewhat more sensitive in the lower normal range. Patients with type 2 are often detected by the constellation VWF:Ag> VWF:RCo, even if both concentrations are in the normal range. The VWF:RCo activity is less sensitive than the collagen binding activity (VWF:CB) for functionally abnormal molecules. However, it can be acutely assayed as a single specific parameter fairly easily by laboratories and thus remains valuable for acute diagnosis. Since it detects the interaction between VWF and the GP Ib receptor, it is an indispensable test for the diagnosis of type 2M.

### 5.1.4. Special diagnostic tests

#### 5.1.4.1. Collagen binding capacity (VWF:CB)

The collagen binding capacity is based on the adhesive functions of VWF, the binding of the molecule to a collagen preparation immobilized on microtiter plates (☞ Figure 5.2).

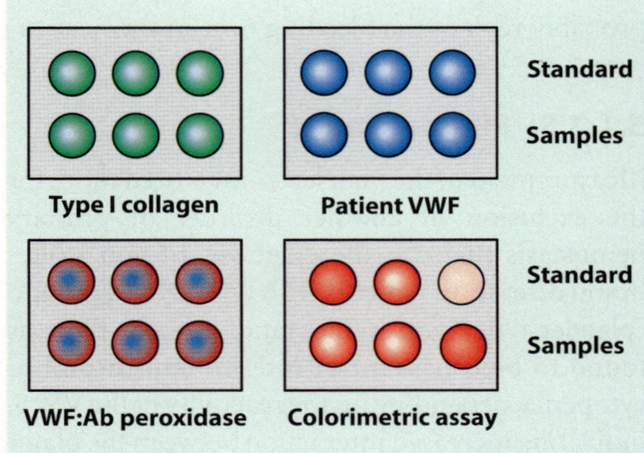


***Figure 5.2:*** VWF: collagen binding assay. A microtiter plate is coated with type I collagen and then incubated with patient plasma. Depending on the collagen binding activity, patient VWF is bound. Binding is detected by means of a peroxidase-labeled antibody and a colorimetric substrate.

In addition to optimally binding collagen (type I and type III), there must be a limited supply. If too many binding sites are available, the competition between fully multimerized VWF and smaller molecules for the available binding sites no longer occurs and the test reflects more the concentration of the VWF:Ag than a functional property. Under optimal conditions, the test reacts in a highly sensitive manner to VWF molecules with loss of large multimers. The parallel assay of VWF:Ag and VWF:CB in the ELISA format from the same dilution and determination of VWF:CB/VWF:Ag ratios provide information about the functional capacity of the VWF. In our laboratory, the limit value is 0.8, i.e. at least 80% of the VWF:Ag must be collagen-binding. All values below this level are pathological and require special investigation with the help of multimer analysis. A disadvantage of the VWF:CB is the high sensitivity to the effects of transport (>24 h at room temperature) and repeated thawing/freezing. Here, we see pathological ratios even if the multimers are unchanged. Due to the difficulty in immobilizing collagen in a lasting manner, commercial tests with type I collagen are not currently available. However, tests with type III collagen are available from two different companies (Progen and Gradipore). The Progen test uses covalently bound collagen. The binding properties of collagen may possibly be altered as a result of this or more collagen may be bound to the plastic surface. Even if the ability to preferentially bind the large multimers is not lost, it is reduced in comparison to type I collagen and to non-covalently bound type III collagen. Generally speaking, the order of preference of functional tests in the detection of large multimers should be as follows: type I > type III (non-covalently bound) > VWF:RCo > type III (covalently bound). The starting material from which the collagen is obtained also plays a role (human placenta, horse tendon). According to studies by Favoloro et al, however, all collagens described in the literature for VWF:CB tests fulfill their purpose.

Measurement of VWF:CB as a single test is of no use. In relation to VWF:Ag, however, a low VWF:CB/VWF:Ag ratio is highly discriminating in detecting a dysfunctional molecule, usually a congenital or acquired loss of large multimers, and rarely an isolated defect of VWF:CB caused by a mutation in one of the collagen binding regions (A3 domain, ☞ below). As a result of the much better inter- and intra-assay precision and the lower variability between different laboratories, the ability to differentiate between a normal and dysfunctional molecule is much better than that of the VWF:RCo.

A further advantage is its response to supranormal multimers. These are detected in the plasma in patients with TTP and after desmopressin infusion. This is thus a practicable method for studying the response to desmopressin .

## 5.1.4.2. Ristocetin-induced aggregation in platelet-rich plasma (RIPA)

The RIPA test is used for identifying an increased or decreased interaction between VWF and the platelet receptor GP Ib. It is conducted with platelet-rich plasma (PRP) from the patient. Thus, it can only be undertaken on the spot and, with great reservation, if sent within 24 hours. It is important to assess not the extent of aggregation following stimulation with a (too high) standard concentration but the threshold value until clear aggregation is triggered (☞ Figure 5.3).

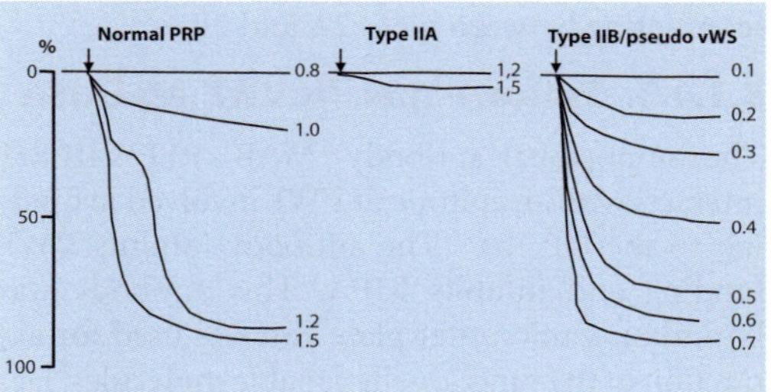


***Figure 5.3:*** Ristocetin-induced aggregation in platelet-rich patient plasma (RIPA test) in patients with type 2A and 2B compared with normal individuals. It is important to use graded ristocetin concentrations (final concentration between 0.1 and 1.5 mg/mL). While all patients with type 2B have increased ristocetin sensitivity, the behavior in type 2A is variable and often cannot be differentiated from that in normal individuals or patients with type 1.

Thus, a low concentration (0.5 mg/mL) should always be used to begin with. The test allows additions of larger quantities into the same aggregation tube. The entire RIPA test can therefore be conducted in PRP of 0.25 to 0.5 mL. Since a laboratory never has sufficient quantities of test material, this possibility is important, especially if small children need to be diagnosed, which is not by any means uncommon in the case of a congenital disease. We have also even performed this test from cord blood without any difficulties.

The sensitivity of the method is too low to make it suitable as a screening test for von Willebrand disease. It is mainly used for identifying patients with increased interaction between VWF and platelets (type 2B and platelet-type von Willebrand disease). The degree of purity of the reagent has increased in recent years. Aggregation with as little as

0.6 mg/mL can still be seen. With 0.5 mg/mL, however, normal individuals no longer show aggregation so this should be the limit concentration for the identification of patients with increased interaction between platelets and VWF.

Hilbert et al showed that patients with type 2M have a decreased RIPA and can be differentiated from type 1 using this test. In the follow-up investigations of patients who were diagnosed as having type 1 using the epitope-specific ELISA (☞ below), Nitu-Whalley et al. found that all patients incorrectly classed as type 1 with a mutation in exon 28 had a greatly reduced RIPA. This means that the RIPA test may have a broader indication than differentiating between types 2A and 2B.

#### 5.1.4.3. Epitope-specific VWF:Ag ELISA

The monoclonal antibody (MAB) RFF-VIII:R/1 interacts with an epitope of VWF involved in binding to the GP Iba. The antibody inhibits VWF binding and inhibits RIPA. This antibody was bound on a microtiter plate and was used for extraction of the functionally capable molecules. Detection was with a polyclonal antibody. While in the first test phase, the laboratory in-house "functional" ELISA test showed encouraging results, the commercial version of the tests did not enable good discrimination between types 1 and 2. There is now a modified test version. However, this modified test is also essentially poorer at detecting patients with type 2 compared with the previously described tests.

#### 5.1.4.4. Botrocetin-induced aggregation in platelet-rich plasma (BIPA)

The snake venom botrocetin induces binding of VWF to GP Ibα but, unlike ristocetin, this binding is independent of the degree of multimerization of the molecule. This allows differentiation between type 2A and 2M. While the reaction with botrocetin is normal in type 2M and abnormal in type 2A, abnormal results are found with both reagents in type 2A. However, BIPA has rather less importance for routine use.

#### 5.1.4.5. Binding studies with isolated platelets

A typical finding in type 2B von Willebrand disease is marked binding of VWF to platelets, often even spontaneously, and at very low ristocetin concentrations. In contrast, the VWF in patients with type 2A does not bind or only at very high ristocetin concentrations. Reduced binding to normal platelets is also found in the platelet-type (pseudo) von Willebrand disease, which is phenotypically very similar to type 2. Conversely, patient platelets bind normal VWF with much higher affinity.

Washed and fixed normal (patient) platelets are mixed with patient (normal) plasma and, to this, increasing concentrations of ristocetin (0-1.2 mg/mL) are added. The test base is allowed to stand for at least 30 minutes at room temperature, Next, the platelets are separated from the plasma and the VWF:Ag not bound to platelets is assayed from the supernatant. Because the test is very laborious, it is only performed by a few specialized laboratories. Platelet-bound VWF can also be assayed by flow cytometry. However, this method currently has no place in routine diagnosis.

#### 5.1.4.6. VWF in platelets

Megakaryocytes are a site of formation of VWF. Provided it is not secreted by platelets into the plasma, it does not come into contact with the VWF-cleaving protease and thus reflects the original synthesized molecule. If platelet VWF can be isolated in the native state, several questions, also of clinical importance, may be answered that remain unanswered from investigation of plasma VWF alone.

The low VWF in blood group 0 is explained by the fact that the plasma half-life is reduced, while the synthesis takes place normally. Hence, a normal platelet VWF in patients with blood group 0 tends to rule out a defect of the VWF gene.

In acquired von Willebrand disease, the VWF is synthesized normally and only changed qualitatively or quantitatively once in the plasma. This often allows differentiation between congenital and acquired forms in clinically unclear situations.

In type 2A in the classic IIA subgroup, 2 mechanisms are known: retention of the large multimers in the Golgi apparatus (group I mutations) and synthesis of a molecule that has increased sensitivity to protease (group II mutations). These may also be differentiated by studying the platelet VWF.

Severe forms of type 1 can also be differentiated from type 3 by the presence or absence of VWF in platelets.

To date, there is unfortunately no standard for platelet VWF and neither are there methods for necessary lysis of platelets nor has a reference unit ($U/10^{11}$ platelets, U/mg protein, % of a platelet pool) been established. There is thus no recognized standard method for the characterization of platelet VWF.

### 5.1.4.7. VW:Ag II (propeptide)

The propeptide is only cleaved after binding has taken place between VWF dimers (multimerization) and secreted together with the mature VWF. It is not influenced by the patient's blood group and does not undergo changes that lead to acquired von Willebrand disease. Assay of the propeptide may thus be very helpful in unclear cases of a bleeding diathesis with changes in VWF. It is assayed in an ELISA system with a specific polyclonal antibody.

At 741 amino acids, the propeptide is unusually large. It is therefore unlikely that it has no biological function. Initial studies suggest that it has modulating properties in inflammatory processes.

### 5.1.4.8. Qualitative changes in VWF

#### VWF multimers

Information about changes in the conformation of the VWF molecule is obtained by studying the multimers. Methods for this were first published by Ruggeri and Zimmerman as well as Hoyer and Shainoff.

Principle of the method: in the Ruggeri and Zimmerman test system, the individual oligomers of VWF are initially separated by electrophoresis in a large-pore agarose gel in the presence of sodium dodecylsulfate (SDS). Affinity-purified $^{125}$I-labeled antibodies to VWF are then allowed to diffuse in and the individual bands are mapped autoradiographically (☞ Figure 5.4).

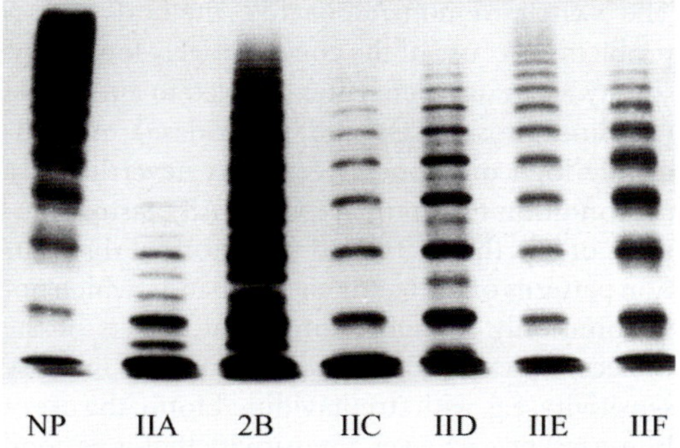


***Figure 5.4:*** Autoradiographic mapping of VWF multimers of various subtypes and subgroups of type 2 VWD compared with normal plasma (NP) in a medium resolution gel. The running direction is from top to bottom (i.e. the large multimers are in the upper part). In normal plasma and plasma from types IIA and 2B, each oligomer consists of a triplet with a central band and an upper and lower subband. The other (sub)types show an abnormal band pattern. Roman numerals indicate subgroups of type 2A.

When using different agarose gels of different concentration in long and short separating distances, gels of low, high and maximum resolution may be obtained.

In recent years, however, radioactive methods have been used less and less often. Moreover, the thickness of the gels of more than 1 mm causes difficulties through extremely long diffusion times during all washing procedures and the necessary incubation with antibodies. The normal run time of these gels is 5 days. It was thus a logical step to simplify the handling of gels through transfer onto suitable membranes (nitrocellulose or nylon). However, method manuals for the different transfer (blotting) techniques treat as "large" any proteins with a molecular weight of a few 100,000 dalton at most. VWF, which is over 10,000 kd, requires special precautions in order to transfer in as quantitative a manner as possible the physiologically important large multimers. Modifications of all known techniques have been described: diffusion, vacuum blot, semi-dry blot and electrotransfer. After trying all variants of these methods, we have found electrotransfer in a chamber that ensures a high, uniform voltage as a result of closely stretched wires to be a reliable method. The phosphate buffer described by Bukh and Ingerslev allows transfer to be undertaken in about 4 hours at currents of 2 amps.

The switch to non-radioactive methods causes problems because of the comparatively lower sensitivity when using enzymes coupled to antibodies (alkaline phosphatase and peroxidase). A sufficiently high dilution of plasma is nevertheless a precondition for optimal results. All plasma dilutions of less than 1:10 lead to abnormal distribution patterns of the bands and subbands, which not uncommonly resemble congenital defects of the molecule. Besides the classic attempts to increase sensitivity, e.g. with streptavidine/biotin, the use of luminescence achieves a sensitivity that is as good as the sensitivity of radioactive methods and even better (☞ Figure 4.2). The short-lived nature of the light reaction has also been improved so that with modern substrates now luminescence persists for more than 24 hours. The move from X-ray film as a medium to videodetection with a highly sensitive CCD camera resulted in the optimum in terms of sensitivity and comfort when evaluating the gels, although at a very high cost price (☞ Figure 5.5). As a result of the optimized mapping of the bands, many more variants can be detected using the CCD camera compared with the time of the X-ray film. The validity of this method can be demonstrated through the detection of specific mutations.

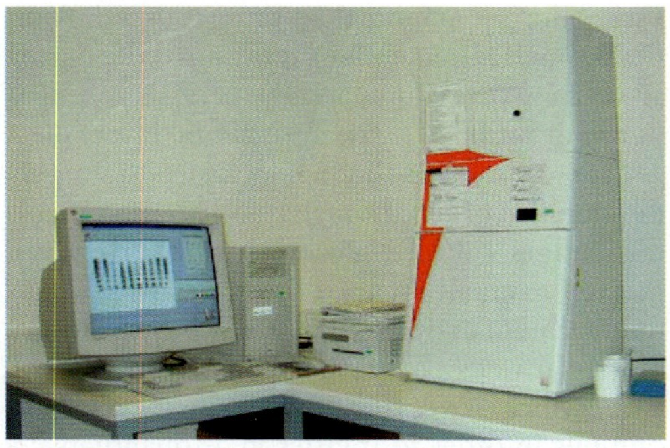

***Figure 5.5:*** Video system for mapping and evaluating luminescent Western blots (Fluorchem®). The CCD camera, cooled to −30°C, is in the upper part of the tower-like light-dense device. The sample space (below) must be sufficiently large to accept a gel.

Nearly all reviews state that at the start of a special investigation the separation of VWF should be in a gel of low resolution. These gels allow the VWF to migrate better than in gels with higher agarose concentrations. This facilitates very good differentiation between samples with loss of the large multimers, supranormal multimers or with a normal picture. However, the variants with an abnormal structure of oligomers commonly seen by us are not really picked up. In order not to miss these, we use a gel of medium resolution as the standard gel. In addition to sufficiently good visualization of the large multimers, structural defects may be recognized to such a good extent that gels of higher resolution are hardly ever needed. Despite the very greatly improved ability to detect a type 2 with the help of the VWF:CB/VWF:Ag ratio, omission of multimer analysis results in most of the type 2 variants not being classified correctly or even missed if there is a normal VWF:Ag. This has been demonstrated in particular by a study of the "von Willebrand Factor" subcommittee of the International Society on Thrombosis and Hemostasis (ISTH). There was a striking difference between the laboratories that worked with a battery of 5 tests and the remainder (81% correct diagnoses vs 31%).

Although the eye is well able to recognize a loss of large multimers or an abnormal quantitative distribution within a lane, a quantitative assessment of the bands is worth striving for. Modern densitometers now allow a comparatively easy assessment of the gels (☞ Figure 5.6).

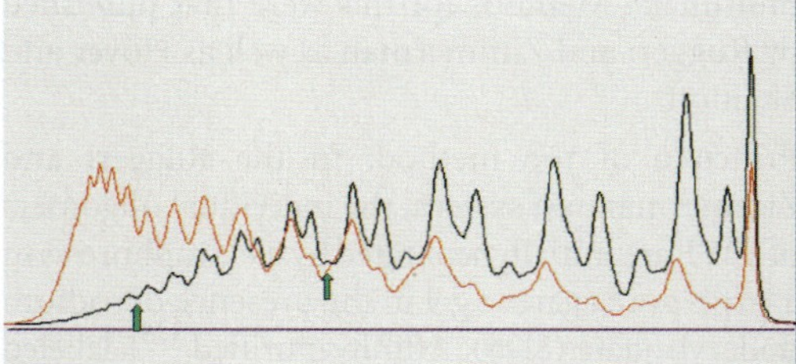

***Figure 5.6:*** Densitometric visualization of VWF multimers in a medium-resolution gel. The running direction is from left to right (i.e. the large multimers are in the left part). Red = normal plasma; black = plasma from a patient with type 2B. The left arrow marks the limit between the large (>10) and medium (6-10) multimers; the right arrow marks the limit between the medium and small (1-5) multimers. The proteolytic changes in the triplet structure are also well visualized.

However, X-ray films have physical properties that greatly complicate densitometric assessment. There are a 100 times fewer gradations of gray between an unexposed (white) and a fully exposed grain of silver (black) than on a light-sensitive microchip. Thus, unexposed and overexposed areas are found much more frequently on an X-ray film than on a microchip. Assessment of these areas leads to incorrect results. Furthermore, there is no consensus as to which are the large, medium and small multimers. The division that we proposed in 1993 is now accepted by most: oligomers 1-5 = small multimers, 6-10 = medium multimers and >10 = large multimers.

### VWF fragments

The proteolytic cleavage that results in regulation of the size of the multimers and the occurrence of the typical triplet (or quintuplet) structure is a physiological process. The fragments that arise can be visualized in a reducing SDS polyacrylamide gel. Variants of type 2 can be subdivided into subtypes with increased (types IIA and 2B) and reduced (subtypes IIC, IID, IIE, IIF) cleavage into fragments. Patients with acquired von Willebrand disease also have increased proteolysis if the acquired von Willebrand disease is a result of thrombocythemia or increased shear stress. However, the current methods are too resource-intensive to be included as part of routine diagnosis.

### FVIII binding capacity of VWF (VWF:FVIIIB)

Using the methods listed so far, mild to moderately severe forms of hemophilia A and type 2N von Willebrand disease cannot be distinguished from each other. However, in some families an additional reduction in VWF:Ag may be observed. Patients with autosomal inheritance of a decrease in factor VIII with normal or additionally decreased VWF are suspicious. The binding of FVIII to the patient's VWF must be measured in order to diagnose type 2.

While the suspicion that there is a FVIII-binding defect of VWF was voiced very early on, it was not until the end of the 1980s that usable methods for laboratory diagnosis were published. The first causal mutations were identified shortly afterward. The first families were discovered in France, especially in Normandy. This defect was thus included in the classification as type 2N (for Normandy). Various test modifications have been described, but they all follow the flowchart shown in Table 5.3 and Figure 5.7.

- The endogenous FVIII is separated from the complex through incubation with high calcium concentrations
- Incubation with a defined quantity of a recombinant FVIII concentrate is then undertaken
- The bound FVIII is either assayed in the chromogenic FVIII test or via incubation with an enzyme-labeled monoclonal antibody to FVIII
- The last step involves measurement of the amount of immobilized VWF and the ratio to bound FVIII is determined (☞ Figure 5.7 and 5.10)

***Table 5.3:*** VWF:FVIIIB test.

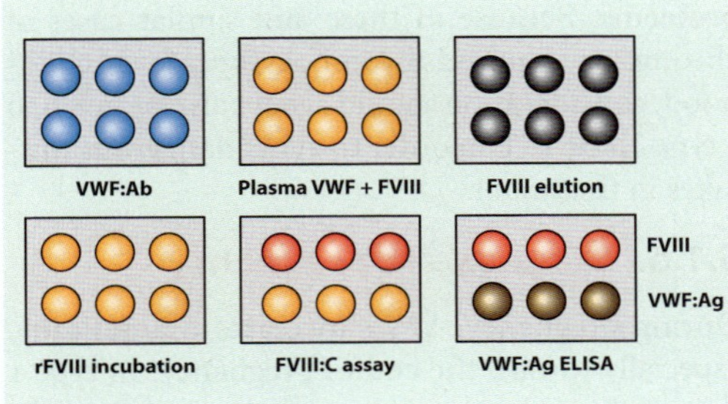


***Figure 5.7:*** Factor VIII binding assay.

Because of the complexity of this test system, assay of VWF:FVIIIB is the preserve of a few specialist laboratories. In a world-wide survey in 1995, 16 laboratories replied that they carry out the test, with 80% of all tests being undertaken in only 4 laboratories.

## 5.1.5. Diagnosis in neonates and small children

Severe type 3 VWD should be easy to diagnose even in neonates because of the absolute deficiency of VWF. For this, the possibility of blood sampling from cord blood or the placenta should be used. In mild forms of type 1, diagnosis in neonates is often difficult since neonates physiologically have a higher VWF level. Furthermore, false-normal levels may also be measured in very excited and screaming children since VWF reacts like an acute phase protein. In order to recognize this situation, a look at the excessively increased VWF:CB is usually sufficient. Only repeated controls help to do this. However, a type 2 form will change into a normal phenotype only in extreme cases. An example of this is the case of a thrombocytopenic neonate. Since the mother was also thrombocytopenic, the attendant physicians suspected a type 2B, which was easily confirmed in the mother using the RIPA test and multimer analysis despite a very high pregnancy-induced VWF:Ag. In contrast, the multimers in the neonate were completely unremarkable and the stress-induced increased parameters VWF:Ag and VWF:CB and the ratio of these were also not diagnostic. The suspected diagnosis was only confirmed by the RIPA test and then, several weeks later, pathological multimers. However, it is extremely difficult to perform the RIPA test in thrombocytopenic neonates given the small amount of blood (about 1 mL) that is available. In this special case, this was achieved without any problems. Because of these and similar cases of chronic or acquired thrombocytopenia in childhood, consideration should always also be given to a type 2B or TTP in order to avoid dangerous mistakes in treatment.

### 5.1.6. Diagnosis in pregnancy

During pregnancy, VWF increases dramatically, especially toward the end of pregnancy. In type 1 this results in diagnostic but not therapeutic problems (normalization) if it is kept in mind that VWF rapidly falls to its original level after birth and late bleeding may then possibly occur. A currently unexplained phenomenon is the fact that about 30% of pregnant women are noted to have loss of the large multimers (Bergmann et al. 1991). This loss does not, however, lead to clinical problems.

## 5.2. Molecular genetic diagnosis

A whole range of genetic defects of VWF are now known to lead to different types of VWD. While in type 1 and type 3, the causal gene defects may be distributed over the entire gene (☞ Figure 3.7), mutation clusters can be localized in specific regions of the VWF gene for some of the other types (☞ Figure 3.9). Thus, mutations for type 2A (phenotype IIA) and type 2B are generally localized in exon 28 of the VWF gene. Defects of FVIII binding are mainly found in exons 18-20. Mutations responsible for VWD 2A (phenotype IIC) are found in the prosequence of VWF. Mutations responsible for VWD 2A (phenotype IID) are localized in exons 50-52 of the VWF gene. In type 3 VWD, only a single mutation is more frequently found. This is a single base deletion (2435delC) in exon 18 of the VWF gene with a high prevalence in Sweden, Poland and Germany (☞ Figure 3.8).

In accordance with the localization of the mutation cluster, limited regions of the gene may be targeted for study in specific VWD subtypes. This is important for rational genetic diagnosis, since study of the VWF gene, because of its 52 exons and size, is otherwise only possible with high outlay of resources. Thus, a condition for molecular diagnosis is that there should always be prior phenotype characterization using conventional methods for investigation of hemostasis. Genetic diagnosis can then confirm the suspected diagnosis. In some cases, a clear classification is only possible through this.

The methods involve the use of all techniques of genetic diagnosis. In order to identify large, especially heterozygous deletions, Southern blot with autoradiography is still in use today. The identification of complete heterozygous deletions is difficult. In these cases, a gene dose assay via densitometry may further help autoradiography compared with a reference gene. PCR-supported gene dose analyses using HPLC are now also used. For polymorphisms of the VWF gene, patients with heterozygous major deletions appear homozygous. The deletion may be concluded to be present if the patient's parents are also available for analysis and if there is apparent non-concordance of haplotypes (☞ Figure 5.8).

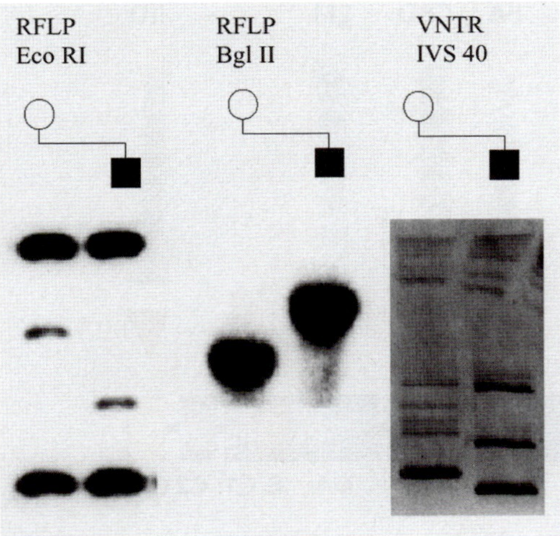


***Figure 5.8:*** Indirect identification of a heterozygous partial deletion of the VWF gene in a patient with type 3 VWD and his unaffected heterozygous mother through analysis of polymorphisms of the VWF gene. The inheritance of the deletion gives the impression of lack of common alleles between mother and son.

Homozygous deletions on the other hand may be easily detected through the absence of amplification products after PCR. A particular problem here is the pseudogene, which is complementary to exons 24-34 of the gene. Even if gene-specific primers are used, amplification may occur and thus lead to false-negative results. The simultaneous running of a reference sample of a patient with a complete homozygous deletion is of great help in differentiating between the gene and pseudogene.

PCR with subsequent analysis of the PCR product through sequencing or restriction enzyme digestion as well as through denaturing HPLC (DHPLC) is a quick and easy-to-perform method for the detection of nearly all point mutations. Since only the coding exons with flanking intron sequences are generally amplified, intron mutations more centrally lying are usually not detected. These mutations can, however, lead to abnormal splicing, which can be detected through study of the VWF mRNA. VWF mRNA can be obtained from platelets for this, and transcribed into cDNA, which serves as the templates for PCR. Analysis of the PCR products is not only able to detect abnormal splicing but moderate deletions, which are not detectable by PCR on genomic DNA, may possibly also be identified through RT-PCR.

Analysis of the entire gene is extremely resource-intensive because of its size and complexity. Exact description of the phenotype enables analysis to be restricted to specific gene regions, but in many patients, especially in those with type 3 or type 1, complete sequencing might be necessary. These comprehensive studies are also facilitated through clever choice of the PCR primers and the simultaneous amplification of all 52 exons in microtiter plates and as a result of progressive automation of sequencing. However, these studies have a very narrow indication for reasons of cost.

Another frequently used strategy is mutation screening using high-resolution gel electrophoresis or DHPLC. Because of the large number of polymorphisms of the VWF gene, these procedures are very difficult to assess. The advantage of lower costs compared with direct sequencing is lost as a result of the subsequent sequencing that is necessary in many exons. Rational genetic diagnosis is thus principally dependent on the exact description of the phenotype.

## 5.3. Phenotype-genotype correlation

Several different subtypes of VWD were described after the introduction of multimer analysis. Until recently, however, there were no data on the prevalence of most of these subtypes. The reason for this is the limited standardization of multimer analysis. Advances in multimer analysis through luminescent visualization combined with electronic image processing (☞ Figure 5.5) and the parallel molecular genetic analysis have allowed extensive phenotype-genotype analyses, which have resulted in interesting correlations and also the clarification of pathogenetic relationships. Thus, defects of post-translational biosynthesis, such as dimerization and multimerization, are responsible for nearly all phenotypes with absence or a relative reduction in large multimers that cannot be attributed to increased proteolysis (☞ Figure 5.9).

### 5.3.1. Defects of dimerization

Dimerization defects are localized in the CK domain at the carboxyterminus of VWF. They are found in some patients with type 3 VWD but

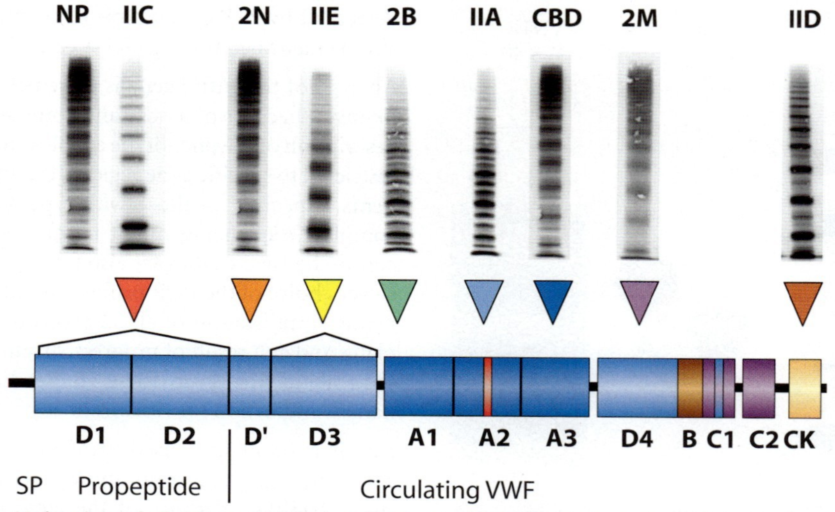


***Figure 5.9:*** Molecular defects in type 2 VWD. Localizations of the different mutations that underlie the subtypes of type 2 VWD and their phenotypes are shown with the relevant multimers. The triangles indicate clusters in the individual domains. Arabic and roman numerals refer to the Sadler (current nomenclature) and Ruggeri (previous nomenclature) nomenclatures, respectively.

mainly in patients with type 2A VWD, subtype IID. In the latter, heterozygous cysteine mutations are present in the CK domain. Multimeric analysis typically shows additional bands between the individual triplets, corresponding to multimers with an odd number of monomers (☞ Figure 5.9).

## 5.3.2. Defects of multimerization

Disorders of further polymerization of the dimers to multimers at their aminoterminal end are caused by two different pathogenetic mechanisms. First, mutations in the D3 domain itself, which contains the cysteines that are directly and indirectly involved in polymerization can prevent or impair multimerization. It is characteristically mainly heterozygous cysteine mutations that are found in these patients. There is usually just a relative reduction in the large multimers, and occasionally also loss of these. Because of reduced proteolysis through the VWF-cleaving protease ADAMTS13, the individual multimers do not have an actual triplet structure but just a broader central band containing subbands close to the actual central band (☞ Figures 4.2 and 5.9). This specific phenotype corresponds to the previous types IIE, IIF and IIH. They are now grouped under type 2A. Mutations outside the D3 domain are only very rarely found. Some homozygous cysteine mutations of the D3 domain have been found in patients with type 3 VWD.

The second pathogenetic mechanism of a multimerization defect is due to mutations in the D1 and/or D2 domain of the VWF propeptide. Each of the two domains that are proteolytically cleaved by the actual VWF contains a CGLC amino acid sequence considered to be a consensus sequence of disulfide isomerase. Both regions apparently have a catalytic role in aminoterminal multimerization. Homozygous or compound heterozygous mutations in the D1-D2 domain are correlated with the phenotype of the former type IIC. This is characterized by lack of the large and occasionally also the medium-sized multimers. A triplet structure is completely absent, indicating greatly reduced proteolysis (☞ Figures 4.2 and 5.9). This phenotype is also included among type 2A. The mode of inheritance is recessive, unlike other type 2A phenotypes. There are evidently also more severe mutations that correlate with a type 3.

## 5.3.3. Increased proteolysis

The regulation of the size of VWF multimers and thus control of the biological activity occurs through proteolytic cleavage between tyrosine 1605 and methionine 1606 in the A2 domain of VWF. Higher sensitivity of VWF to its specific protease ADAMTS13 correlates with specific mutations in the VWF A2 domain. The result is increased proteolysis with loss of the large and medium-sized VWF multimers and thus loss of the biological activity in primary hemostasis. In some cases, a reduced VWF:Ag is also found. In each case, however, the ratio of functional activity, measured as VWF:RCo or VWF:CB to VWF:Ag is clearly decreased. The multimers are seen as more intense subbands in the triplet structure of the oligomers, which are also a product of the increased proteolysis (☞ Figure 4.2).

### 5.3.4. Increased affinity for GP Ib

Mutations in the region of the VWF-GP Ib binding site at the start of the A1 domain lead to a constitutionally increased affinity for platelet GP Ib, resulting in platelet agglutination triggered by acute phases or even spontaneous agglutination of platelets. Besides the consumption of platelets and the associated thrombocytopenia, there is loss of high-molecular-weight VWF multimers. Multimeric analysis does not allow this type, also termed 2B, to be differentiated from type 2A with increased proteolysis (☞ Figure 4.2). However, this may be done with ristocetin-induced platelet aggregation at low ristocetin concentrations. All mutations may be found in the above region. Hence, a clear classification is also possible through genetic diagnosis.

### 5.3.5. FVIII binding defect

The VWF-FVIII binding defect or type 2N VWD may not in some situations be differentiated from hemophilia A. The reason for this is, in the classic case, the isolated FVIII binding defect without other changes in VWF. Many cases of so-called "female hemophilia A" are in fact this type. The majority of the mutations are found in exons 18, 19 and 20 of the D' domain of VWF. "More severe" mutations have been described that are associated with FVIII activities of as little as 1% and a "milder" mutation in exon 20 with FVIII:C around 20%. In addition to the VWF:FVIII binding assay (☞ Figures 5.7 and 5.10), the diagnosis may also be made through gene analysis.

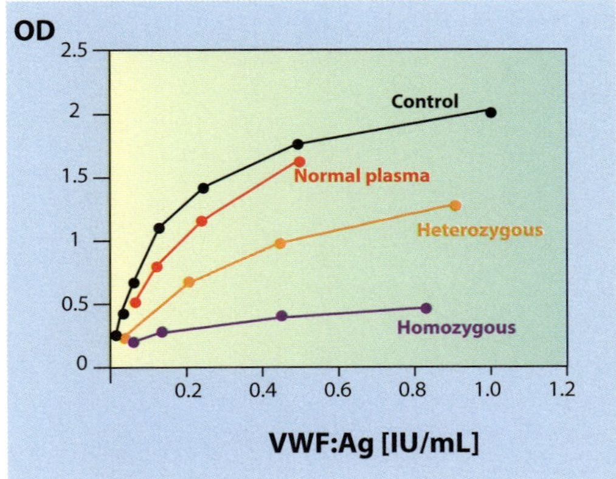


***Figure 5.10:*** Relationship between VWF: FVIIIB and the genotype at different concentrations of the VWF:Ag. With increasing concentration of VWF, the binding of FVIII (visualized as optical density (OD) on the y axis) increases in normal plasma and normal control plasma until saturation. Heterozygous individuals for a type 2N mutation show the same behavior, but at a lower level (≈ 50% binding capacity). In contrast, VWF:FVIIIB is not present in patients with type 2N (homozygous) or is drastically reduced. The increase with higher VWF:Ag levels is also absent or only minimal.

### 5.3.6. Other variants

Although mutations have already been described for type 2M, to date no specific mutation cluster has been identified. In one variant of a type 2A VWD where there is a distorted structure of the triplets in addition to a relative loss in large multimers, cysteine mutations are mainly found, but again without a distinct cluster.

# Acquired von Willebrand Syndrome (VWS)

# 6. Acquired von Willebrand Syndrome (VWS)

The first description of an apparently acquired form of von Willebrand disease (VWD) dates back to 1968. Simone and colleagues described the occurrence of a severe bleeding tendency in patients with systemic lupus erythematosus. At that time, VWF could not be assayed. However, the prolonged bleeding time in the presence of normal platelet counts and reduced FVIII activity very closely resembled the findings in patients with congenital VWD. The next four patients, who were described by Ingram and colleagues in 1971, also had immunological disease. In the years that followed, more and more diseases were described that were associated with acquired VWD, designated today as von Willebrand Syndrome (VWS).

Several papers also discuss this disease. They are, however, restricted to existing case reports, since even large coagulation departments do not have sufficient patient numbers to provide a rounded picture of this disease that is considered to be rare. There is a clear tendency to publish clinically severe cases rather than mild bleeding complications. Thus, there is a predominance of patients with lymphoproliferative disorders, for instance, who nevertheless only represent a minority in the population of patients with acquired VWD.

Our coagulation laboratory in Hamburg has been working for more than 15 years with more than 100 doctors in the German-speaking countries and over this time has increasingly attributed unexplained bleeding complications to initially unsuspected acquired VWS. As a result of this, the attendant physicians have become attuned to this disease with the result that we are seeing a clear increase in referrals with this suspected diagnosis. In 2001 and 2002, 25% of all patients with VWS had an acquired form. This chapter, which contains a description of conditions that may be accompanied by acquired VWS as well as a critical comparison with the literature and data from a retrospective survey from 1998 and 1999, aims to increase awareness about this condition.

In 2001 and 2002, we studied 5,069 plasma samples from patients whose history or current symptoms suggested a disorder of primary hemostasis. Of these samples, 1,209 (24%) had VWD and 306 patients from this group (25%) were diagnosed as having acquired VWS on the basis of the results available. What was striking was that while 80% of patients with congenital VWD did not come from the Hamburg area, the great majority of patients with acquired VWS (74%) were from Hamburg and the surrounding region. This suggests that these patients had acute bleeding problems that had to be investigated by a local laboratory. Compared with data from 1998 and 1999 that had already been published, there was no significant change, so there was a stable picture over a 5-year period.

For correct classification, we recorded data from the medical history as far as possible. However, for laboratories that are involved as the secondary referral center, this is inevitably difficult. Hence, about 20% of patients ultimately cannot be correctly classified and must be disregarded in the statistics. Specific methods included VWF:Ag (latex method in acute cases), VWF:RCo (also in acute cases) and subsequently VWF:CB and multimer analysis in a low-resolution system. Furthermore, factor VIII activity was assayed in fresh samples. Whenever possible, the RIPA test was also performed without discovering a case with an increased RIPA. A decreased RIPA also tends to be uncommon. Measurement of the VWF:Ag in platelets proved useful in differentiating from congenital VWD. Whenever an immunological etiology has to be considered, investigations for antibodies against VWF are indicated (☞ Table 6.1). However, current tests usually yield negative results.

| Direct methods |
|---|
| • Test analogous to the Bethesda test for detecting FVIII inhibitors (VWF:RCo, VWF:CB, VWF:Ag)<br>• Direct binding of antibodies to VWF on immobilized VWF<br>• A disadvantage is the strong background when using anti-human IgM, which is less with anti-human IgG, because blood group antigens are an integral part of the VWF molecule even if VWF from subjects with blood group 0 is used<br>• Adsorption of the immune complex on a solid phase (protein A Sepharose)<br>• Protein A binds VWF directly. False-positive results are therefore to be expected if suitable negative controls are not run at the same time<br>• Acquired hemophilia A must be excluded through a Bethesda test |
| Indirect methods |
| • Response of VWF to DDAVP, factor VIII/VWF concentrates and/or high-dose IV immunoglobulin IgG<br>• Diagnosis of the primary disease and disappearance of acquired VWS after successful treatment of the primary disease |

***Table 6.1:*** Special tests for the diagnosis of acquired VWS. Tests for the identification of antibodies to the FVIII/VWF complex.

## 6.1. Pathophysiological mechanisms

In most patients with acquired VWS, VWF is synthesized in normal and, not uncommonly, even increased concentrations and released into the plasma. The reduction or qualitative changes occur in the plasma as a result of different pathophysiological mechanisms typical of the relevant diseases (☞ Table 6.2). In some patients, however, the pathophysiological mechanism cannot be determined.

| Specific or non-specific autoantibodies that lead to immune complex formation and increased elimination of VWF |
|---|
| • Lymphoproliferative diseases<br>• Neoplasms<br>• Immunological diseases |
| Adsorption of VWF onto malignant cell clones or other cell surfaces |
| • Lymphoproliferative diseases<br>• Neoplasms<br>• Myeloproliferative diseases<br>• Pathological shear stress |
| Increased proteolysis of VWF |
| Specific |
| • Myeloproliferative diseases<br>• Pathological shear stress<br>• Uremia<br>• Ciprofloxacin |
| Non-specific (plasmin) |
| • Primary hyperfibrinolysis<br>• Secondary hyperfibrinolysis<br>• Thrombolytic therapy |
| Pathological shear stress |
| • Congenital heart diseases<br>• Aortic stenosis<br>• Endocarditis<br>• Vascular malformations (Osler's disease, Kasabach-Merritt syndrome)<br>• Severe arteriosclerosis<br>• β-Thalassemia |
| Reduced synthesis |
| • Hypothyroidism |
| Unknown |
| • Valproic acid<br>• Viral diseases<br>• Hepatic disease |

***Table 6.2:*** List of the pathogenetic mechanisms involved in the different diseases.

### 6.1.1. Lymphoproliferative diseases

This group accounts for a significant portion of patients both in the literature (30%) and in the registry (48%). However, these figures are in contrast to our data with only 29 patients (12%) in the period 2001/2002. Nevertheless, these few patients (16 with a monoclonal gammopathy of uncertain clinical significance [MGUS] of the IgG type and 6 of the IgM type) had the most prominent symptoms. One patient with gastrointestinal hemorrhage required more than 20 packs of blood/week.

In no patient were we able to detect circulating antibodies to VWF. Our standard method for detecting antibodies is analogous to the Bethesda test for FVIII (☞ Table 6.1). The direct measurement of bound immunoglobulins on immobilized VWF would probably have provided positive results much more frequently. In all patients, VWF was clearly decreased and in the patient with MGUS of the IgG type it was dysfunctional (acquired type 2). In contrast, the patients with a paraprotein of the IgM type had acquired type 1. The different types correlating with the immunoglobulin class were also found in all other years. This tallies with most literature data but is in sharp contrast to the data from Milan (Federici and coworkers). In these patients, the massive bleeding problems are striking and even investigational methods for a bleeding diathesis are virtually always remarkable. Thus, the diagnosis is nearly always made and hence the overrepresentation in the literature is easily explained. It is important to determine whether the bleeding tendency has in fact started late in life. If only phenotypical data are available, some of the patients may easily be classified as having congenital type 2A (subtype IIE), since multimer analysis provides very similar results (☞ Figure 6.1).

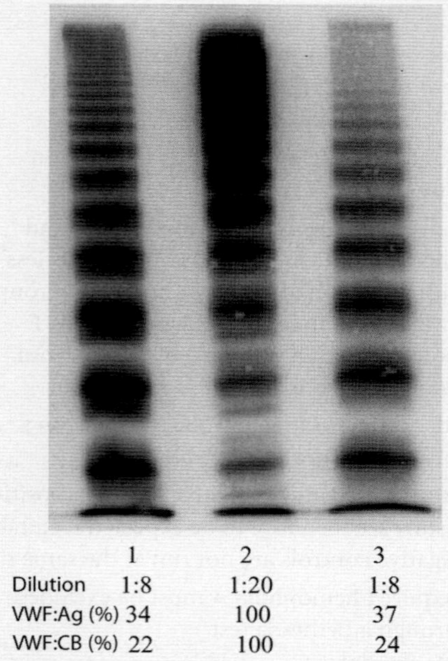


***Figure 6.1:*** Comparison of VWF multimers of a patient with MGUS of the IgG type (#1) with those from normal pooled plasma (#2) and those from a patient with congenital type 2A (IIE). Without knowledge about the history, it is not possible to differentiate between a congenital and an acquired form of VWD. In both patient samples, the large multimers are present but the concentration of these is greatly reduced.

Patients with a paraprotein of the IgM type show an unmistakable multimeric pattern (☞ Figure 6.2). The giant VWF-IgM complexes destroy the agarose during their passage through the gel and sometimes even leave holes. A brief inspection of the gels is thus sufficient for the correct diagnosis.

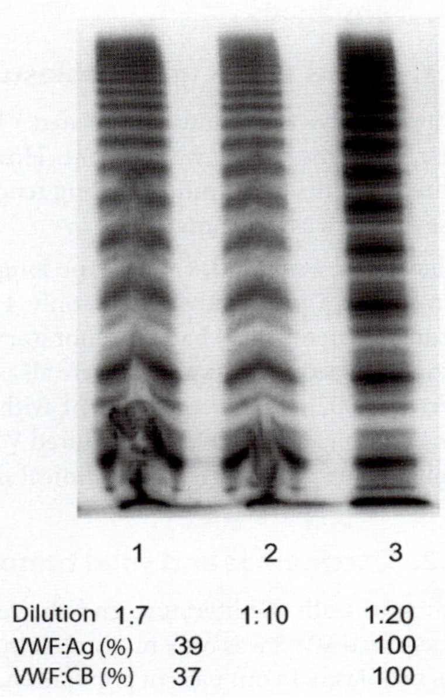


***Figure 6.2:*** Comparison of the VWF multimer of a patient with MGUS of the IgM type (#1, 2) with those from normal pooled plasma (#3). All multimers are present (acquired type 1). However, the greatly distorted band structure is a striking feature and is typical of an IgM paraprotein.

## 6.1.2. Thrombocythemia

This group represents the second largest number of patients in the literature (18 %) and in the registry (15 %). Our figure of 33% is higher. However, not all patients investigated in our laboratory had bleeding but were investigated to confirm the diagnosis or to know what action to take in the future. Thus, the higher patient number can be easily explained.

Thrombosis and bleeding, not uncommonly at the same time, are frequent complications in myeloproliferative diseases. Whereas thrombosis is the dominant feature in primary thrombocythemia, patients with polycythemia rubra vera and especially osteomyelofibrosis tend more to have hemorrhage.

Hemorrhage manifest itself mainly as gastrointestinal bleeding, followed by mucosal bleeding and intra- or postoperative hemorrhagic complications. Bleeding may also be prominent during dental procedures. Nosebleeds are also common. Skin hemorrhage is described as hematomas, ecchymoses and bruises. Petechiae are never seen. This spectrum of bleeding symptoms is very similar to the spectrum seen in congenital VWD. The mean platelet count in 100 patients from the literature was 2,050 ± 1,107 x $10^9$/L at the time of bleeding. The two contrasting disorders of hemostasis - bleeding and thromboembolism - do not occur at all stages of the disease but depend on the platelet count. If the platelet count is less than 1,000 x $10^9$/L, thromboembolism is very much the dominant feature, while bleeding clearly predominates at counts above 2,000 x $10^9$/L. Between 1,000 and 2,000 x $10^9$/L both complication may occur, and not uncommonly may even be simultaneous (☞ Figure 6.3).

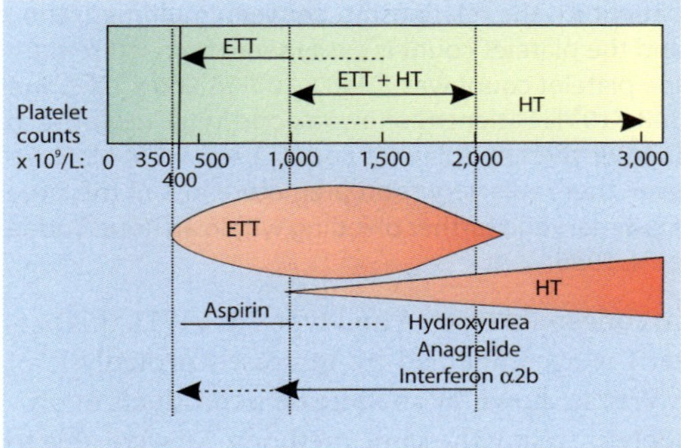


***Figure 6.3:*** Relationship between clinical symptoms and the platelet count (based on Michiels JJ). Below a count of 1,000 platelets/nL thrombotic complications clearly predominate (ETT = erythromelalgic/thrombotic thrombocythemia). Spontaneous hemorrhage occurs mainly at platelet counts of more than 1,500 x $10^9$/L and is the main clinical symptom at counts of more than 2,000 x $10^9$/L (HT = hemorrhagic thrombocythemia). Between 1,000 x $10^9$/L and 2,000 x $10^9$/L, the picture is mixed and thromboembolism and hemorrhage not uncommonly occur simultaneously. ASS is able to prevent the thromboembolic complications but potentiates the bleeding symptoms or even triggers them. Based on Michiels et al, 2001, with permission.

Apart from the thrombocythemia, investigation of hemostasis reveals a prolonged bleeding time, a normal concentration of FVIII:C and VWF:Ag and a disproportionate reduction in VWF:RCo and VWF:CB. The large multimers nearly always show an absolute or relative reduction. In very rare cases, an acquired type 1 was seen. In addition to the loss of the large multimers, there is a prominent fastest subband if the individual oligomers are separated into triplets (☞ Figure 6.4).

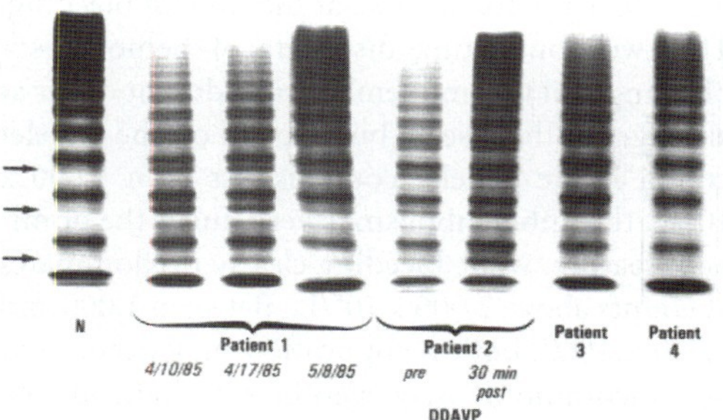


***Figure 6.4:*** VWF multimers in 4 patients with primary thrombocythemia in a medium-resolution gel. In patient #1, the relationship between multimerization and the platelet count is easily seen; from left to right the platelet count was 2,240 x $10^9$/L; 1,960 x $10^9$/L and 348 x $10^9$/L. Patient #2 shows a good initial response to DDAVP therapy (platelet count 2,760 x $10^9$/L). However, there was very soon premature loss of the large multimers and further bleeding within an hour. Budde et al. 1986.

In congenital type 2A and type 2B VWD, this pattern is accompanied by increased proteolysis of VWF, as shown by an increase in products of proteolysis. Using the same methods, we were able to demonstrate that this is also the case for patients with myeloproliferative diseases. The demonstration that increased physiological cleavage is involved was achieved by using fragment-specific monoclonal antibodies.

### 6.1.3. Reactive thrombocytosis (RT)

Although the large VWF multimers are also reduced in reactive thrombocytosis (RT) depending on the platelet count, hemorrhagic complications occur only very rarely, if at all. Compared with patients with thrombocythemia, the VWF:Ag is much higher (acute phase reaction) and can compensate for the loss in large multimers as a result. Moreover, the increase in the platelet count is of comparatively short duration and the changes in VWF are completely reversible with the decrease in the platelet count. In contrast to myeloproliferative disorders, platelet function is also normal, although this only plays a marginal role in myeloproliferative disorders. Patients with RT are also treated with ASS much less often.

### 6.1.4. Neoplasms

#### 6.1.4.1. Wilms tumor (nephroblastoma)

In most case reports of tumor-associated VWS in children, a Wilms tumor was present. However, only three patients had a mild bleeding tendency, while seven were asymptomatic.

After the disease was cured, VWS was no longer demonstrable. In a prospective study, only 4 of 50 consecutive patients (8%) had the laboratory constellation of an acquired VWS, but were all asymptomatic. In 2002, we saw one patient with mild bleeding complications. Overall, acquired VWS in nephroblastoma probably has little clinical significance.

#### 6.1.4.2. Carcinomas and solid tumors

According to both the literature and the registry (5%), acquired VWS was only rarely seen in other types of neoplasm. In our patient population, there were only three patients with carcinomas and one associated acquired VWS with mild symptoms.

### 6.1.5. Immunological diseases

The first descriptions of patients with acquired VWS concerned patients with systemic lupus erythematosus (SLE) and autoantibodies to VWF. Since VWF is a giant molecule with many immunogenic structures, it is theoretically a logical target protein in immunological diseases. In practice, however, autoantibodies to VWF are rare compared with autoantibodies to FVIII, which is also a large glycoprotein and even a few powers of ten less common than autoantibodies to platelet membrane components. In the literature, only 15 cases are described, usually in association with SLE (6 patients) and autoimmune diseases of another etiology (6 patients) and very rarely in mixed connective tissue disease (1 patient), graft versus host disease (1 patient) and in Ehlers-Danlos syndrome. The registry contains only 4 patients with autoimmune diseases and in our patient population autoimmune diseases were reported in three cases.

### 6.1.6. Cardiovascular diseases

In our study, patients with cardiovascular disease represent a major group (39%). Although acquired VWS in cardiac defects was described as early as 1986, since then only a few cases have been published. It could thus be a laboratory phenomenon of low clinical importance. Only for patients with aortic stenosis and gastrointestinal bleeding was it demonstrated that a functionally abnormal VWF was responsible for the bleeding. One reason why this pathogenetic mechanisms is not considered for unexplained hemorrhagic complications in often elderly patients is the high, and sometimes very high, concentration of VWF, especially during acute bleeding (☞ Figure 6.5).

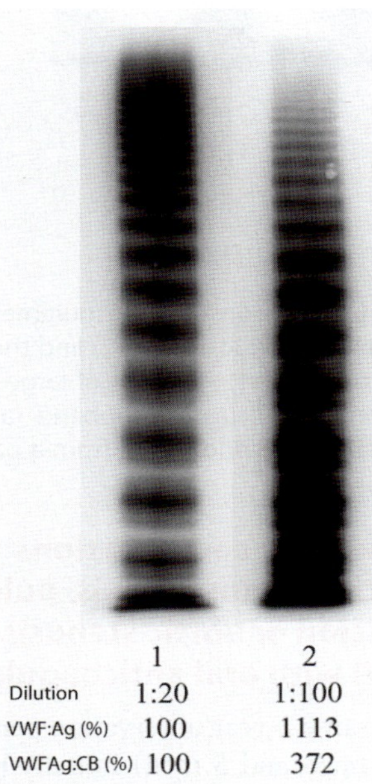


***Figure 6.5:*** Comparison between VWF multimers in a female patient with aortic stenosis and an ovarian tumor (#2) and VWF multimers from normal pooled plasma (#1). The (relative) loss of the large multimers is clearly seen. Although VWF:Ag was very greatly increased, the patient had severe gastrointestinal and gum bleeding.

Since all parameters of VWF (antigen and functional markers) exceed the normal range, the functional deficiency of this is overlooked if not all parameters are titrated separately and the ratio of functional parameters to the concentration is not studied. Since the functional defect of VWF in cardiovascular diseases arises as a result of an acquired loss of large multimers, the VWF:CB is, next to multimer analysis, currently the most sensitive test for detecting this loss. The ratio of VWF:RCo and VWF:Ag theoretically provides the same information but here the poor reproducibility of the VWF:RCo should be borne in mind, especially at high levels. The parameters VWF:Ag and VWF:RCo, which are rapidly available, as well as VWF:CB, which cannot usually be assayed on a daily basis, have almost 100% sensitivity for loss of the large multimers if performed correctly, but should be complemented by multimer analysis with quantitative densitometry. Most of these patients will require several invasive procedures over the years so correct diagnosis is very important.

With increasing age, arteriosclerotic processes occur that progressively narrow the vessel lumen in the arterial vascular tree. The increased shear stress that arises as a result of this induces two chronic changes in VWF with opposite effects. First, there is an increased concentration of VWF. It increases from the age of 40 by about 0.06 U/mL every 10 years. In the acute stage of diseases and in chronic diseases, this increase may be excessive. Through its stabilizing function for FVIII, a high VWF is always also accompanied by a high FVIII level. This means an increased risk of venous thrombosis. An increase in risk for arterial thromboembolic complications as a result of high VWF levels is less well documented but appear plausible. Second, the loss of large multimers induced by shear stress nevertheless means a danger of bleeding as a result of a disorder of primary hemostasis. This often silent defect of primary hemostasis not uncommonly manifests itself if in addition there is a second defect (e.g. of secondary hemostasis). Thus, patients who require oral anticoagulation after a heart valve replacement or after venous thrombosis unexpectedly develop life-threatening cerebral hemorrhage shortly after the start of anticoagulation.

## 6.2. Clinical situations where patients with cardiovascular diseases are at special risk

### 6.2.1. Unexpected bleeding complications during surgical procedures in patients with advanced arteriosclerosis and aortic stenosis

Over a 2-year period, 14 patients were found to have acquired type VWS during investigations for diffuse intraoperative bleeding. Gastrointestinal operations were involved in all cases. These patients were usually elderly, with a median age of 72 years (48-87 years). Most (8) had peripheral arteriosclerosis, 5 had clinically significant aortic stenosis and one patient had both.

Of the laboratory results obtained, an increased VWF:Ag (median 2.85 U/mL) and a normal but relatively reduced VWF:CB (median 1.85 U/mL) suggested acquired type 2 VWS. This was confirmed in all cases by subsequent multimer analysis. When investigating this type of bleeding it is important to determine the exact concentration of the antigenic and functional properties of VWF. By determining the ratio, cases where further investigation is necessary will be identified. Here it is especially important to bear in mind that in all of our cases where defective VWF was not the cause of the bleeding complication, the ratio was high (usually >2). This can easily be explained by the stress-induced secretion of supranormal multimers from the storage organelles. It is thus particularly striking that in all the above patients the ratio was much lower (<0.8).

### 6.2.2. Bleeding complications in patients with endocarditis

Over the course of two years, samples from 4 patients with severe bleeding complications in the context of endocarditis were sent to our laboratory. In 2 cases, the aortic and mitral valve were both affected. In one case, the shear-stress-induced disturbances of bleeding components were so severe that the symptom complex of thrombocytopenia, hemolytic anemia with schistocytes and massive cerebral symptoms suggested TTP. However, the cerebral symptoms came about not as a result of thromboses but recurrent cerebral hemorrhage. The situation was only normalized after surgical removal of the affected valve. The shear-stress-induced loss of large multimers seen in this patient was also observed in the remaining patients (☞ Figure 6.6). A further striking feature was the very high, usually excessively high, VWF. The greatly increased bleeding tendency that has long been recognized (anticoagulation is contraindicated in these patients) is thus explained by an acquired type 2 VWS.

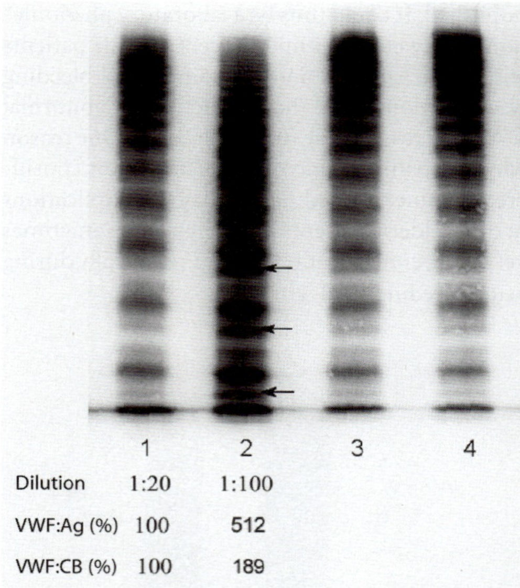


***Figure 6.6:*** Comparison of VWF multimers of a female patient with endocarditis (#2) and those of normal pooled plasma (#1). The loss of large multimers and the pronounced, fastest subband (arrows) are clearly seen. Lanes #3 and #4 are from a patient with normal VWF.

### 6.2.3. Bleeding complications in patients with arteriosclerosis, pulmonary hypertension or aortic stenosis during treatment with oral anticoagulants

During the same 2-year observation period, 9 patients (4 women and 5 men) initially had unexplained bleeding complications during treatment with oral anticoagulants. In all cases, the INR was in the target range and the bleeding was observed during the initial period of anticoagulation. The most severe symptoms were cerebral hemorrhage in 5 patients resulting in death or very severe handicap. The indication for the anticoagulant treatment was aortic valve replacement (2 patients), pulmonary hypertension (1 patient) and atrial fibrillation (2 patients).

In these patients, too, the VWF:Ag was clearly raised in nearly all (1.33-3.55 U/mL, mean 2.28 U/ml) and the VWF:CB was disproportionately low (0.69-2.43 U/mL, mean 1.01 U/mL). The ratio between the VWF concentrations was thus clearly abnormal (ratio 0.27-0.79, mean 0.65). All patients had an absolute or relative loss of large multimers. After all common defects of primary hemostasis had been excluded, the conclusion was that acquired VWS was the only or principal cause of the catastrophic bleeding complications. While the disorder of hemostasis had previously been tolerated more or less without symptoms, the additional disorder of plasma hemostasis as a result of oral anticoagulants contributed to the severe hemorrhage.

In addition to these extremely threatening complications, a further 4 patients (2 with cardiac failure and 2 with atrial fibrillation) developed such severe bruising that the oral anticoagulation had to be stopped. After the switch to low-molecular-weight heparins at a prophylactic dose (dose as for high-risk patients), the bleeding improved but one female patients still needed 1 to 2 blood transfusions per week even on this therapy.

If it is assumed that approximately 3% of the elderly population have clinically silent aortic stenosis, the number of patients at risk for the complications described above is very high. Even though most cases of bleeding as a result of acquired VWS follow a benign course, it is nevertheless surprising that little attention is paid to this mechanism, and the literature on this subject is rather meager.

Children with congenital heart defects, especially with shunt diseases and stenoses, are also at risk of bleeding. Even in the case of a patent ductus arteriosus, a prospective study found acquired type 2 VWS in 25%. In all cases, the pressure gradient was also particularly high and patients were usually picked up just on auscultation.

## 6.3. Acquired von Willebrand Syndrome in patients with different diseases

This group of patients is heavily represented in the literature (approximately one third of cases), is found much less frequently in the registry and for our patients the figure is somewhere in between. Four diseases in 61 patients (78%) account for the most common primary conditions in this group, based on the literature: treatment with valproic acid derivatives or hydroxyethyl starch, hypofunction of the thyroid gland and hemoglobinopathies. In contrast to this, acquired VWS in these diseases was seen only rarely in both the registry and in our patient population. Thus, the cases described were probably mostly mild VWF deficiency states without dysfunction (acquired type 1) and more a laboratory phenomenon than a clinical problem. Many more patients with disturbances of clotting would otherwise be picked up, particularly as the diseases or drug treatments are common. In order to investigate the discrepancy between the literature and clinical reality during treatment with valproic acid, three German pediatric clinics participated in a prospective study with 50 patients over a 2-year observation period. Although VWF:Ag markedly fell in all patients, in no case did it drop below the low normal level of 50%. Since epileptic children are often in an acute phase stage, the fall in VWF:Ag after treatment is easily explained. This study found that although acquired type 1 VWS during treatment with valproic acid does occur, these are isolated cases and it is not a general problem. The cause of the bleeding diathesis that is undoubtedly present in these patients probably needs to be investigated in relation to other components of the system of hemostasis (e.g. thrombocytopenia).

Acquired VWS in patients with uremia is also a controversial subject. We encounter this about to two to three times a year. A problematic issue is that the greatly increased VWF makes effective therapy difficult.

During our work with other centers, we increasingly noted that viral diseases, principally chronic hepatitis C, was clearly overrepresented as a cause of acquired VWS (☞ Table 6.3).

Up to that point, the literature contained only one report of a patient with Epstein-Barr virus infection. The observed symptoms of a tendency to hematomas, epistaxis and intraoperative bleeding are typical of primary hemostasis. Like patients with cardiovascular problems, the patients were usually older, the VWF:Ag was greatly increased (typical of patients with hepatic diseases), the VWF:CB to VWF:Ag ratio was reduced and the large multimers were absent or relatively decreased (☞ Table 6.4). A dysfunctional protein is thus clearly involved (acquired type 2). Besides patients with chronic hepatitis C, we regularly see patients with hepatic diseases of other etiology and acquired type 2 VWS. Whether, as it appears to be, acquired VWS in the course of hepatitis C infection is a problem of older patients or whether the bleeding tendency found in all patients is only seen in

| Primary disease | Registry (n=186) | Literature (n=266) | Hamburg (n=246) |
|---|---|---|---|
| Lymphoproliferative | 89 (48) | 79 (30) | 29 (12) |
| Monoclonal gammopathy of uncertain significance | 43 (23) | 37(14) | 22 (9) |
| Multiple myeloma | 16 (9) | 19 (7) | 4 (2) |
| Waldenström's disease | 8 (4) | 5 (2) | 3 (1) |
| Non-Hodgkin's lymphoma | 8 (4) | 10 (4) | 0 |
| Hairy cell leukemia | 0 | 1 | 0 |
| Acute lymphatic leukemia | 1 | 0 | 0 |
| Myeloproliferative | 29 (15) | 48 (18) | 82 (33) |
| Essential thrombocythemia | 21 (11) | 17 (6) | 71 (29) |
| Polycythemia rubra vera | 1 | 9 (3) | 5 (2) |
| Chronic myeloid leukemia | 5 (3) | 22 (8) | 1 |
| Myelofibrosis | 2 (1) | 0 | 4 (2) |
| Reactive thrombocytosis | 0 | 0 | 1 |
| Neoplasms | 9 (5) | 15 (6) | 4 (2) |
| Wilms tumor | 0 | 11 (5) | 1 |
| Carcinomas and solid tumors | 9 (5) | 3 (1) | 3 (1) |
| Peripheral neurectodermal tumor | 0 | 1 | 0 |
| Immunological | 4 (2) | 15 (6) | 3 (1) |
| Systemic lupus erythematosus | 0 | 6 (2) | 1 |
| Autoimmune diseases | 4 (2) | 6 (2) | 2 (1) |
| Mixed connective tissue disease | 0 | 1 | 0 |
| Graft-versus-host disease | 0 | 1 | 0 |
| Cardiovascular | 39 (21) | 31 (12) | 95 (39) |
| Congenital and acquired cardiac disease | | | |
| Multiple or not defined | 24 (13) | 0 | 38 (15) |
| Ventricular septum defect | 0 | 10 (4) | 6 (2) |
| Atrial septum defect | 2 (1) | 1 | 1 |
| Aortic stenosis | 7 (4) | 5 (2) | 21 (9) |
| Mitral valve prolapse | 2 (1) | 10 (4) | 0 |
| Endocarditis | 0 | 0 | 4 (2) |
| Patent ductus arteriosus | 0 | 0 | 2 (1) |
| Pulmonary hypertension | 0 | 0 | 13 (5) |
| Other | | | |
| Angiodysplasia | 4 (2) | 5 (2) | 0 |
| Ehlers-Danlos syndrome | 0 | 1 | 0 |
| Generalized arteriosclerosis | 0 | 0 | 10 (4) |

| Primary disease | Registry (n=186) | Literature (n=266) | Hamburg (n=246) |
|---|---|---|---|
| Miscellaneous | 16 (9) | 78 (28) | 33 (13) |
| Drugs | | | |
| Ciprofloxacin | 0 | 2 (1) | 0 |
| Griseofulvin | 0 | 1 | 0 |
| Valproic acid | 1 | 19 (7) | 3 (1) |
| Hydroxyethyl starch | 0 | 11 (4) | 0 |
| Infectious | | | |
| Hydatid cyst | 0 | 1 | 0 |
| Epstein-Barr virus infection | 1 | 1 | 0 |
| Hepatitis C | 0 | 0 | 5 (2) |
| Other systemic | | | |
| Hypothyroidism | 3 (2) | 21 (8) | 0 |
| Diabetes | 0 | 7 (3) | 0 |
| Uremia | 6 (3) | 3 (1) | 7 (3) |
| Hemoglobinopathies | 2 (1) | 10 (4) | 1 |
| Sarcoidosis | 1 | 0 | 0 |
| Telangiectasia | 1 | 0 | 0 |
| Ulcerative colitis | 1 | 0 | 0 |
| Hepatic diseases | 0 | 0 | 13 (5) |
| Myelodysplastic syndrome | 0 | 0 | 3 (1) |
| Idiopathic | 1 | 1 | 1 |

***Table 6.3:*** Diseases that are associated with acquired von Willebrand Syndrome. Modified from Budde et al. 2002.

| Associated illnesses | Lympho-proliferative 29 (12) | Myelo-proliferative 82 (39) | Cardio-vascular 95 (39) | Miscella-neous 40 (16) | Total 246 (100) |
|---|---|---|---|---|---|
| VWF:Ag (U/dL, median)<br>range | 47<br>9-307 | 99<br>48-342 | 124<br>35-524 | 194<br>14-1120 | 123<br>9-1120 |
| VWF:CB (U/dl, median)<br>range | 17<br>4-160 | 62<br>23-366 | 84<br>35-364 | 124<br>18-440 | 80<br>4-440 |
| VWF:CB/VWF:Ag ratio (median)<br>range | 0,44<br>0.11- 1.22 | 0,66<br>0.37-1.08 | 0,72<br>0.28-0.97 | 0,63<br>0.38-1.48 | 0,67<br>0.11-1.48 |
| Loss of large multimers (%) | 76 | 97.6 | 100 | 90.9 | 95.1 |
| Positive anti-VWF antibodies versus test patient samples * | 0/7 | n.t. | n.t. | n.t. | 0/7 |

***Table 6.4:*** Laboratory findings in our patients with acquired VWS. * Measurement of the residual concentrations of VWF:Ag and VWF:CB after mixing with normal plasma. n.t. = not tested. Based on Budde et al. 2002.

advanced age rather than in adolescents or young adults needs to be clarified by prospective studies in younger patients with hepatitis C infection. The pathophysiological mechanism of acquired VWS in hepatitis C infection is not currently known. However, chronic hepatitis C infection is known to lead to immunological diseases, e.g. immune thrombocytopenia and acquired inhibitory hemophilia.

The results of the international survey at large centers, the observations in our current patient population and the search of the literature have clearly shown that acquired VWS may be expected to occur in some not uncommon diseases. Thus, if unexpected bleeding occurs in these patients, acquired VWS should be considered. It is obviously clear that this problem is underestimated. However, large prospective studies to confirm this are lacking. Since the theoretical number of possible patients with acquired type 2 VWS is very high (☞ above), such a study is also interesting for companies that produce drugs for the treatment of VWD (concentrates or DDAVP).

# Treatment of von Willebrand Disease

# 7. Treatment of von Willebrand Disease

The different treatment options for patients with VWD will depend on the clinical severity, risk of bleeding, e.g. during surgery, and the type of VWD. Patients with VWD 1, the most common diagnosis, only rarely require prophylaxis. In many cases, local treatment, such as a pressure bandage at the site of bleeding, is sufficient. Systemic prophylaxis or treatment may be necessary in patients with mild VWD, e.g. during major surgery or surgery in regions that cannot be adequately controlled or where local treatment is not possible. This applies in general for tonsillectomy, adenectomy and urogenital surgery.

Two main treatment options are available for patients with VWD (☞ Table 7.1). When used, the special points listed in Table 7.2 should be considered.

| Type 1 | Type 2 | Type 3 |
|---|---|---|
| • DDAVP<br>• Tranexamic acid<br>• (FVIII/VWF) | • FVIII/VWF<br>• Tranexamic acid<br>• (DDAVP) | • FVIII/VWF<br>• Tranexamic acid<br>• (Platelet concentrate) |

***Table 7.1:*** Treatment and prophylaxis of von Willebrand disease. Controls: VWF:RCo, (FVIII:C).

| | |
|---|---|
| Type 3 | DDAVP is ineffective |
| Type 2B | Caution with DDAVP |
| Type 2N | DDAVP ineffective in severe cases |
| Type 2A IIC Miami | FVIII/VWF possibly not sufficient (rFVIIa) |

***Table 7.2:*** Special points to be kept in mind in the treatment of von Willebrand disease.

The first therapeutic approach uses the secretion of endogenous VWF from the storage organelles (Weibel-Palade bodies, ☞ Figure 3.3), while the second therapeutic option consists of replacement of VWF using appropriate plasma preparations. These must contain a sufficient quantity of biologically active VWF.

The additional administration of an inhibitor of fibrinolysis (tranexamic acid) may be beneficial.

## 7.1. Desmopressin (DDAVP)

DDAVP improves hemostasis by increasing the plasma levels of FVIII and VWF. It can thus be successfully used in the treatment of patients with mild hemophilia A and VWD 1. After administration of DDAVP, the bleeding time becomes shorter and the plasma levels of FVIII and VWF rapidly increase. They reach their maximum within the first hour and then fall over 4 to 8 hours. The rise in FVIII and VWF:Ag reaches approximately 3 to 4 times the baseline level. The increase that is achieved is striking, especially the increase in the high-molecular-weight multimers, and thus especially the biological activity of VWF in primary hemostasis (☞ Figure 7.1).

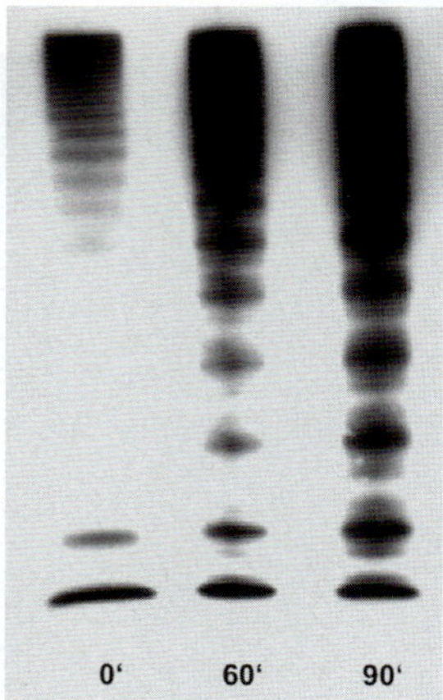


***Figure 7.1:*** Action of DDAVP at a dose of 0.3 µg/kg body weight in a patient with type 1 VWD. Clear rise in VWF:Ag after 60 and 90 minutes.

This is also seen as an overproportionate higher increase in VWF:RCo and VWF:CB (☞ Figure 7.2) in relation to VWF:Ag. DDAVP may be used in patients with type 1 VWD for dental procedures or minor surgery and bleeding episodes. It is now generally accepted that a DDAVP test to assess the efficacy of DDAVP should always be undertaken in type 1 VWD and never undertaken in type 3 because of the a priori lack of efficacy. The successful use in many cases including type 2 has led to the suggestion that these patients should also be tested accordingly. The use in VWD types 2A, 2M and 2N can thus be considered.

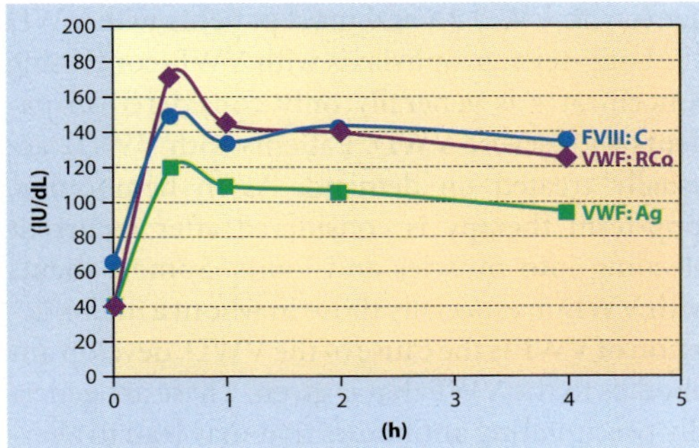


***Figure 7.2:*** Typical time course of the VWF parameters after administration of DDAVP in a patient with type 1 VWD. The VWF:RCo shows an overproportionately higher increase.

However, the efficacy very much depends on the subtype (☞ Figure 7.3 and 7.4). The use in type 2B continues to be controversial because of the possible thrombocytopenia associated with it. Some type 2B patients have, however, been successfully treated with DDAVP.

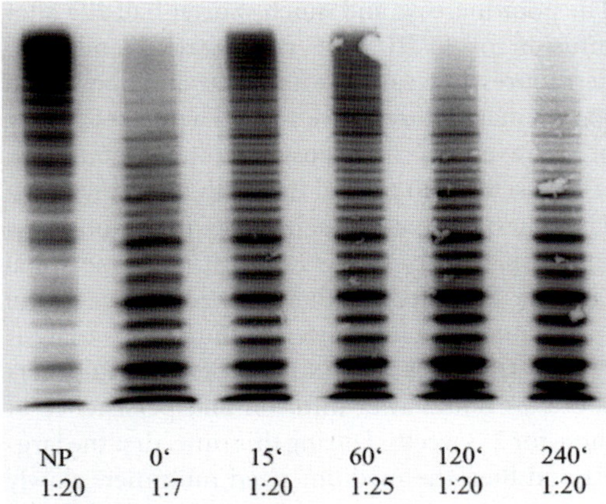


***Figure 7.3:*** DDAVP effect in a patient with type 2A VWD. Compared with the pattern before DDAVP infusion, more large multimers were found and the VWF:Ag increased by a factor of 2.5 but there was no normalization of the large multimers and the VWF:CB/VWF:Ag ratio remained pathological. After 4 hours, the concentration of large multimers had fallen to the initial level, while the VWF:Ag was still above the initial level.

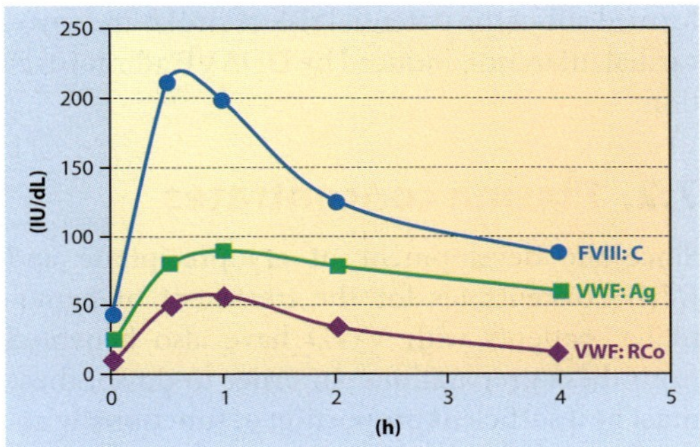


***Figure 7.4:*** Time course of the VWF parameters after administration of DDAVP in a patient with type 2A VWD with increased proteolysis (phenotype IIa). While the VWF:Ag and especially FVIII:C show a good increase, the increase in the VWF:RCo is unsatisfactory. Overall, the duration of effect should be regarded as unsatisfactory.

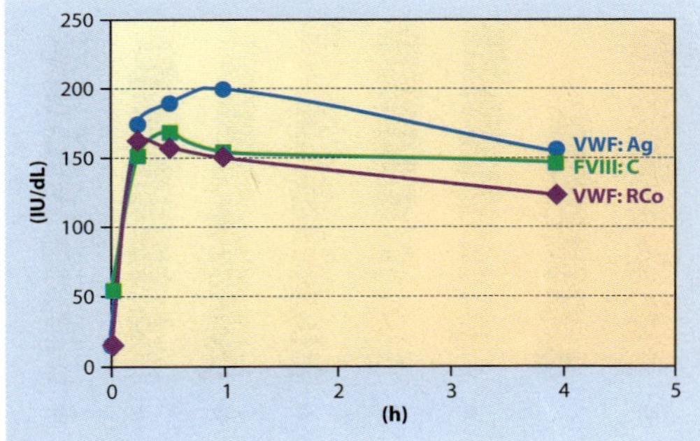


***Figure 7.5:*** Time course of VWF parameters after administration of DDAVP in a patient with type 2M VWD. VWF:Ag, VWF:RCo and FVIII:C show a good increase. However, VWF:RCo shows an increase that is proportionately slightly less than VWF:Ag, indicating a functional defect of VWF/GP Ib binding; the duration of effect may be considered satisfactory.

More frequent use of DDAVP is associated with a reduction in effect (tachyphylaxis). This is due to emptying of the storage organelles that first need to be replenished. Repeat administration of DDAVP earlier than 8 hours after the first administration is thus less effective.

Sudden facial flushing and transient headache may occur as side effects of the treatment. Especially in small children, there may be water retention, associated with hyponatremia. DDAVP can trigger seizures, particularly in specially predisposed patients (relative contraindication: history of cerebral seizures). Older patients (>60 years) should be informed about the potential risk of stroke and myocardial infarction induced by DDAVP administration.

## 7.2. Plasma concentrates

Since the development of cryoprecipitate and FVIII concentrates for the treatment of hemophilia, patients with VWD have also benefited from these preparations. In order to do so, there must be a sufficient proportion of functionally active VWF in these preparations. In particular, the large multimers, which are particularly active in primary hemostasis, must be present in a suitable concentration. Thus, some degree of quality control may be obtained through analysis of multimers and the collagen binding activity in the concentrate (☞ Figure 7.6).

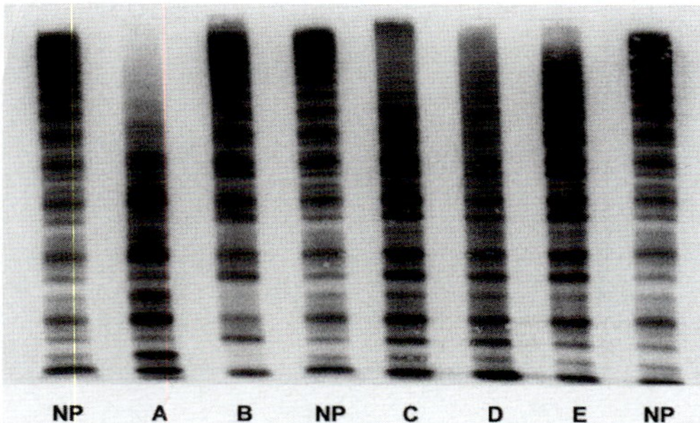


***Figure 7.6:*** Multimeric analysis of five FVIII/VWF concentrates of different manufacturers. Most concentrates show a reduction in the large multimers and not uncommonly an altered triplet structure. Because of the presence of high-molecular-weight VWF multimers, preparation B appears particularly suited.

With the development of increasingly purer products for the treatment of hemophilia A, e.g. recombinant FVIII concentrates, only few preparations are unfortunately now available for the treatment and prophylaxis of VWD.

Only plasma concentrates containing VWF may be considered for the prophylaxis and treatment of VWD 3. Patients with VWD 3 have complete absence of VWF; thus, no VWF can be released from stores. DDAVP will thus have absolutely no effect in these cases. In many cases of VWD 2, the only promising approach is again substitution with plasma preparations. This applies especially to patients with severe forms of VWD 2N, many patients with VWD 2A and most patients with VWD 2B. Long-term prophylaxis with VWF-containing concentrates is generally only considered in patients with severe VWD. Patients with VWD2 are usually treated on demand. As in hemophilia, long-term therapy is considered after recurrent bleeding into muscles and joints. Some patients with VWD 3, especially those in whom a major deletion of VWF is the cause of the VWD, develop antibodies to the VWF that is given. These are generally precipitating antibodies that may lead to allergic reactions, immune complex disease and nephrotic syndrome with continued administration. Inhibitor elimination therapy, as in hemophilia A, is thus associated with the corresponding risks.

## 7.3. Treatment of acquired von Willebrand Syndrome

### Lymphoproliferative diseases

The poor increase and much shorter half-life after infusion of FVIII/VWF concentrates and after desmopressin treatment has been described in 36 representative cases since 1977. The successful use of intravenous high-dose immunoglobulin G (IVIGG) has also proved its worth for many years. The best outcomes are achieved with monoclonal gammopathies of the IgG type. If no monoclonal IgG can be detected, the prospect of successful treatment is much lower. Multimeric analysis demonstrated the reappearance of large multimers about 24 hours after infusion and persistence of these for 2-3 weeks. During this time, first the largest and then the medium-sized multimers slowly began to disappear. In no case was a cure achieved. However, the period of recovery was virtually always sufficient for surgical interventions. The time of 48 hours until normalization can be shortened to about 24 hours using higher doses (1 g/kg body weight). As soon as IVIGG has been administered, the shortened half-life is seen to a much lesser extent. Thus, initial IVIGG infusion followed by FVIII/VWF concentrates is a rapid-acting therapeutic option. In the IgM type, IVIGG is without effect. Symptomatic treatment is thus the only possibility here. With successful treatment of the primary disease, the acquired VWD in lymphoproliferative diseases disappears. On the other hand, uncontrollable bleeding is an indication for recombinant factor VIIa.

## Thrombocythemia

Bleeding can be stopped using both FVIII/VWF concentrates and DDAVP infusion. Normalization of VWF may, however, result in thromboembolic complications. Moreover, correction lasts for much shorter than in congenital VWD. This is especially the case after DDAVP infusion. Thus, if severe bleeding complications occur, cytoreduction is indicated. After normalization of the platelet count, the hemorrhagic diathesis disappears even though the functional impairment of platelets remains unchanged. That the continuing impairment in platelet function is of little clinical significance is demonstrated, amongst other things, by the fact that it has no effect on the prognosis. In the acute case with excessive thrombocythemia (in our case, the count was more than 6,000 x $10^9$/L), plateletpheresis can halve the counts very rapidly and may be life-saving (☞ Figure 7.7).

## Reactive thrombocytosis (RT)

Bleeding complications are not to be expected with reactive thrombocytosis. We have never experienced a case of this ourselves and to our knowledge the literature has not so far described any such cases. In the unlikely event that this scenario occurs, the measures described above are effective.

## Neoplasms

### ▶ Wilms tumor (nephroblastoma)

Based on available reports, most patients are without symptoms. The remaining 30% have only mild symptoms that can easily be controlled with DDAVP without any problems. After successful treatment of the primary disease, the acquired

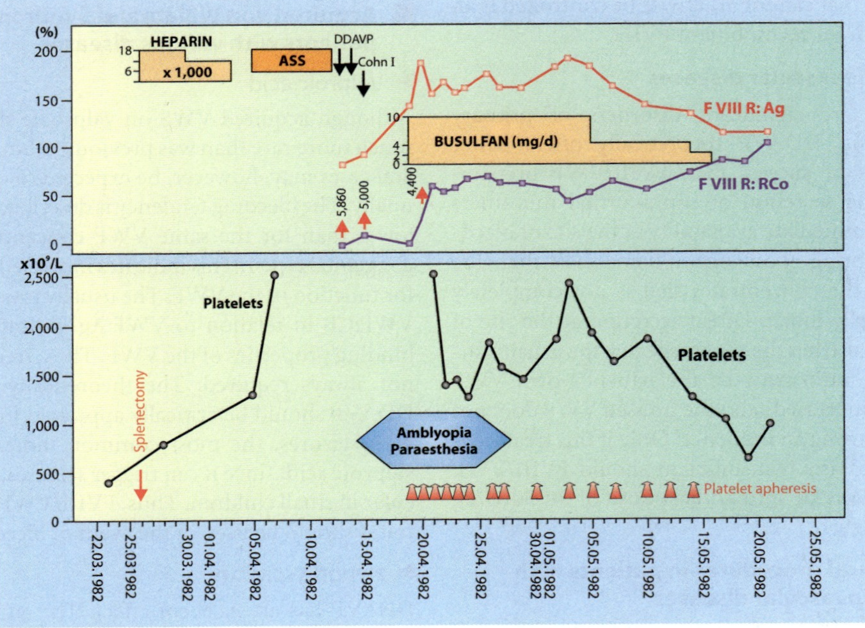


***Figure 7.7:*** A patient with polycythemia rubra vera, at the time aged 29 years, required splenectomy because of an atraumatic rupture. Following this, the platelets underwent a massive increase to over 6,000 x $10^9$/L and first heparin and then acetylsalicylic acid therapy was initiated. On the 9th postoperative day, the patient had severe bleeding from the abdominal incision and was referred to us for investigation of his clotting. Analysis showed type 2 von Willebrand Syndrome. The bleeding time was very prolonged and platelet aggregation greatly impaired. Short-term hemostasis was achieved using the vasopressin analogue DDAVP. However, definitive hemostasis was only achieved after infusion of Cohn's fraction 1. Two days later, the patient noticed severe paresthesia and had increasing blindness without any neurological and ophthalmologic changes being visible. In order to achieve a rapid reduction in his platelet counts, we initiated combined therapy with cytopheresis and cytostatics (busulfan). A complete remission was achieved with this within 3 weeks.

VWS could no longer be detected in all published cases.

#### Carcinomas and solid tumors

In these patients mild forms also predominate. Thus, DDAVP is also the drug of choice here. Although not many cases have been reported, acquired VWS nearly always disappeared following successful treatment.

### Immunological diseases

Whenever an autoantibody has induced acquired VWS, the symptoms are severe. Since DDAVP-secreted or infused VWF is very rapidly broken down, both therapeutic options frequently fail. It is typically the case that the acquired VWS usually persists even after successful treatment of the primary disease. Successful use of IVIGG is possible but there are hardly any case reports about this. Immune adsorption is theoretically an option. Bleeding that cannot otherwise be controlled is an indication for recombinant FVIIa.

### Cardiovascular diseases

If there are significant disorders of primary hemostasis, DDAVP theoretically offers better prospects of success than FVIII/VWF preparations. The secretion of supranormal multimers and the immediate availability at the site of bleeding can bring about better hemostasis than the VWF of the concentrates that is not completely functionally intact. Direct secretion at the site of bleeding also has the advantage that the usually unfavorable ratio between the patient's own VWF (usually increased) and the infused VWF does not have so strong an influence. Only if this treatment for hemostasis is insufficient should FVIII/VWF preparations be infused at a dose of 30-50 U/kg body weight.

### Surgical procedures in patients with cardiovascular diseases

If bleeding cannot be controlled by the measures described above, recombinant FVIIa is another option.

### Bleeding complications in patients with endocarditis

The abnormal ratio between the patient's own VWF and infused VWF is here often particularly unfavorable because of the greatly increased VWF:Ag, and the danger of bleeding is commonly extreme. Thus, early consideration should be given to the possibility of using recombinant FVIIa.

### Bleeding complications during treatment with oral anticoagulants

On the one hand, rapid normalization of the vitamin K-dependent factors through PPSB is important in severe hemorrhage and, on the other, vitamin K administration to consolidate the effect. If it is possible to wait for a few hours for an effect to occur, vitamin K administration alone is sufficient. After consolidation of acute hemorrhage, the future anticoagulant therapy needs to be reappraised. If the potential danger from vitamin K antagonists outweighs the benefit, a trial of low-molecular-weight heparins in the upper prophylactic range is a possible alternative. However, bleeding may also be expected here. In this case, the lack of an antidote and the long half-life are clear disadvantages.

### Acquired von Willebrand Syndrome in patients with various diseases

#### Valproic acid

Although acquired VWS on valproate therapy is much more rare than was previously thought, several cases may, however, be expected to occur annually. The bleeding tendency is described as being lower than for the same VWF concentration in congenital type 1. This indicates increased capacity for function of the VWF. The usually much higher VWF:CB in relation to VWF:Ag indicates better binding properties of the VWF. Thus, treatment is not always required. The theoretically effective DDAVP should be critically appraised in patients with seizures, the most common indication for valproic acid, since it can trigger seizures, in particular in small children. Thus, FVIII/VWF concentrates should be used in the event of bleeding.

#### Hypothyroidism

DDAVP has an excellent effect. The administration of thyroxine as treatment of the primary disease leads to complete normalization as a result of increased protein synthesis. Hence, acquired VWS in hypothyroidism is only a secondary clinical problem.

#### Uremia

As in cardiovascular diseases, there is usually always an unfavorable ratio between the patient's own VWF and infused VWF, which does not result in such a great effect. Thus, DDAVP often offers better chances than FVIII/VWF concentrates, for the considerations outlined above. Corresponding studies were published as early as the start of the 1980s. The favorable effect of conjugated estrogens (Presomen) has also been repeatedly described. Moreover, dialysis results in a marked normalization of hemostasis even though it is not always sufficient.

### ▶ Hepatic diseases

The same criteria apply as for patients with uremia. However, Presomen has not been shown to be effective in these patients and is not recommended.

# Thrombotic Thrombocytopenic Purpura (TTP)

# 8. Thrombotic Thrombocytopenic Purpura (TTP)

The VWF multimer size after secretion from endothelial cells is regulated by the specific VWF-cleaving protease ADAMTS13. A reduction in the protease to <10% or complete absence of it leads to persistence of so-called supranormal multimers, which are highly reactive. Since VWF has the property of an acute phase protein, increased secretion from endothelial cells during infections or other processes in individuals with congenital or acquired deficiency of ADAMST13 can trigger the formation of thrombi in the microcirculation and lead to the clinical picture of thrombotic thrombocytopenic purpura (TTP). Even today, this is still associated with a high morbidity and significant mortality.

The clinical picture originally described by Moschcowitz in 1924 is characterized by the generalized appearance of hyaline thrombi in the microcirculation, while the related hemolytic uremic syndrome (HUS), especially in childhood, mainly affects the kidney in most cases. Besides platelets, the hyaline thrombi found in TTP principally contain VWF, while in disseminated intravascular coagulation the thrombi almost exclusively contain fibrinogen and fibrin and hardly any VWF. A distinction was made early on between a hereditary and an acquired form of TTP. In both forms, there is deficiency of ADAMTS13, caused by mutations of the ADAMTS13 gene in the hereditary form, and by antibodies to ADAMTS13 in the acquired form in most cases. It was, however, shown that deficiency of ADAMTS13 with subsequent TTP can also occur in malignant diseases, after bone marrow transplantation and following the use of platelet aggregation inhibitors (ticlopidine, clopidogrel). The difference between the various forms is very important in relation to the prognosis, the treatment to use and genetic counseling. Although an antibody to the protease can be demonstrated using plasma exchange (Bethesda method) in many TTP patients with the acquired form, this is evidently not always reliable, as experience has shown. Thus, identification of antibodies during the course of the condition may be negative, despite ongoing deficiency of ADAMTS13. In these patients, a correct diagnosis is therefore not always possible. In all hereditary cases, however, there is a high likelihood that mutations of the ADAMTS13 gene will be found. Thus, gene analysis allows differentiation between the hereditary form and an acquired form even in cases where conventional diagnostic techniques are insufficient.

## 8.1. Conventional methods of diagnosis

TTP is easy to recognize in the presence of all symptoms described by Moschcowitz (☞ Table 8.1). These include petechial hemorrhage because of thrombocytopenia, hemolytic anemia, fever, acute renal insufficiency and neurological symptoms. However, TTP must also be considered in patients with a mild clinical course or in the absence of one or more symptoms. In children, the diagnosis of ITP or Evans syndrome is often made although investigations for the corresponding autoantibodies are negative and the disease has a more severe course than is otherwise the case. In particular, if an infection is the trigger for TTP, the disease is interpreted as infection-associated ITP. However, even adults with undetectable protease activity and antibodies to the protease can sometimes recover surprisingly quickly without specific treatment and have often been discharged home before we have been able to give the result of the ADAMTS13 assay. There are now several assays available for identifying ADAMTS13 deficiency (☞ Table 8.2).

- Petechiae
- Hemolytic anemia
- Fever
- Acute renal failure
- Neurological symptoms

***Table 8.1:*** Pentad of symptoms in classic TTP, as originally described by Moschcowitz. Presentations with only very few symptoms (e.g. only thrombocytopenia) are also possible.

### 8.1.1. Detection of supranormal multimers

As early as 1983, Moake et al. observed that, especially in the symptom-free period, VWF multimers that were much larger than usual were found in the plasma (☞ Figure 8.1).

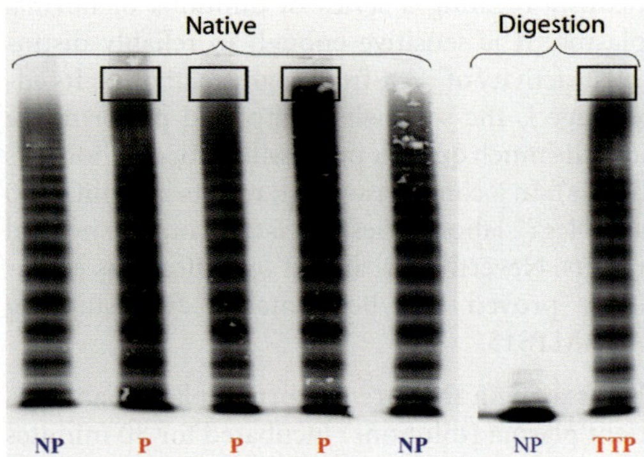


***Figure 8.1:*** Supranormal VWF multimers (framed) in the plasma of patients with TTP in remission compared with normal plasma (VWF multimers are underdigested by the protease present in the sample after activation).

They reached the size of multimers in platelets, usually disappeared in the acute phase and later reappeared. Moake concluded from this that VWF must normally be processed in the plasma by proteolysis in order to prevent spontaneous adhesion and aggregation. Despite attempts at identifying this protease, which initially appeared similar to calpain, it was not until almost 15 years later that it could be detected in functional tests and it took a few years more before it could be characterized exactly. In addition to supranormal multimers, a noticeable feature in the complete absence of the protease is that the typical triplet structure is almost completely lacking. Given the possibility of specifically detecting the protease in functional tests, the methods to detect multimer changes are only of secondary importance.

## 8.1.2. Assay of the activity of ADAMTS13 based on Furlan et al.

In 1996 and 1997, Furlan and coworkers published a test method that today remains the gold standard for all assays of the activity of this protease. A purified cryoprecipitate is used as the substrate. It is important that only fractions that contain high-molecular-weight VWF but no protease activity are added to the separating column. Other proteases that can non-specifically cleave VWF are inactivated by an inhibitor of serine proteases. Since VWF in its native form cannot be cleaved by ADAMTS13, it must be transformed into a denatured form, thereby exposing the cryptic cleavage sites. The denaturing is achieved by using a special buffer with low ionic strength and 1.5 M urea. Even in this buffer, the cleavage of VWF takes place only very slowly. Thus, the protease in the plasma to be studied is activated by $BaCl_2$. After activation, the diluted plasma sample is mixed with the substrate. The mixture is carefully placed on a cellulose acetate plate that swims as a dialysis membrane on the buffer. After 24 hours of incubation, the cleavage of VWF is complete and the mixture is harvested from the membrane and inactivated by EDTA. Multimer electrophoresis of the cleaved VWF then takes place (☞ Figure 8.2).

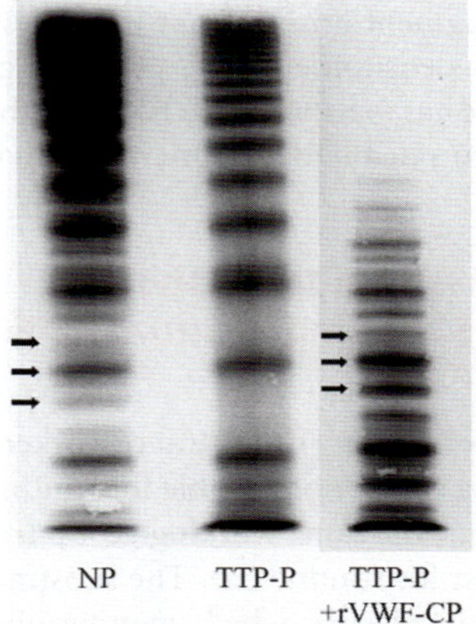


***Figure 8.2:*** Effect of recombinant ADAMTS13 on plasma from a patient with TTP. NP = normal plasma with normal triplet structure; TTP-P = plasma from a patient with TTP; a noticeable feature is lack of a triplet structure in the absence of an effect of the protease. By adding recombinant ADAMTS13, proteolysis occurs with loss of the large multimers and generation of triplets.

This test is quantitative by simultaneously performing a dilution sequence. It is sensitive enough to reliably differentiate activity of 1% from activity of <1%. Its disadvantage is that only a few specialized laboratories can perform it and that it takes 3 days for a result.

By assaying a mixture of normal plasma and patient plasma (dilutions) incubated at 37 °C for 30 minutes, inhibitors of the protease can be detected and quantified using the Bethesda test for clotting factors.

### 8.1.3. Assay of the activity of ADAMTS13 based on Tsai et al.

At the same time as Prof. Furlan's working group, Tsai et al developed and published details of a test that is at least as or even more laborious to perform. Instead of dialysis in a denaturing buffer, treatment with guanidine hydrochloride is used. Using VWF treated in this way as the substrate, test plasma dilutions are incubated. After completion of incubation, the VWF is separated in an SDS-PAGE gel and, after transfer onto a membrane, incubated with an antibody to VWF. Detection is undertaken using a radioactively labeled antibody against the former antibody. The conditions are selected such that the amount of dimer from the 176 kd fragment arising from proteolysis can be measured densitometrically. According to Tsai himself, he has to measure each sample three times in order to reliably determine the activity of the protease.

### 8.1.4. Assay of the activity of ADAMTS13 using residual VWF:CB and VWF:RCo

The test devised by Furlan and coworkers is time-consuming and is not suitable for routine laboratories. Thus, the same working group tried to develop a test for routine use. The substrate used is fresh frozen plasma, which may be obtained in large quantities from blood banks. ADAMTS13 and serine proteases are inactivated by incubation with EDTA and Pefabloc®. Removal of EDTA and change of conformation is achieved by dialysis in the buffer above with low ionic strength. The substrate is then divided up into aliquots and frozen. Immediately before use, concentrated urea is added so that a final concentration of 1.5 M is achieved. Since less substrate is contained in the starting material, the endogenous VWF of the plasma being tested has to be extensively cleaved before the test mixture is incubated. Thus, the protease in the plasma being studied is activated for 30 minutes instead of 5 minutes with BaCl2. Thereafter, the diluted plasma sample is mixed with the substrate. The mixture is incubated for 2 hours at 37 °C. The cleavage of VWF is then so far advanced that VWF:CB is much reduced. The mixture is inactivated by adding sulfate ions. The VWF:CB is then assayed using immobilized collagen type III. This test gives a quantitative result by simultaneously running a series of dilutions of normal plasma. It is sensitive enough to reliably distinguish activity of <3% from higher activities. Its advantage is the somewhat simplified performance and the much quicker processing (about 6 hours vs 5 days). In a comparison test, results in 3 out of 30 samples (2 laboratories) deviated from the normal results. Nevertheless, all test modifications examined proved to be suitable for studying ADAMTS13.

By assaying a mixture of normal plasma and patient plasma (dilutions) incubated for 30 minutes at 37 °C, inhibitors of the protease can be detected and quantified using the Bethesda test for clotting factors.

The test has been modified by us and the Baxter laboratory in Vienna in such a way that recombinant VWF is used as the substrate. This has the advantage of using native non-proteolyzed VWF.

A further modification consists of a prolonged incubation period and assay of the residual VWF:RCo. The results tallied well with the Furlan test apart from the fact that the lower limit of detection was 6%.

### 8.1.5. Assay of the activity of ADAMTS13 using fragment-specific monoclonal antibodies

The ELISA method developed by Obert et al is very elegant. The substrate used is recombinant VWF added to a quantity of 80-100% of a plasma standard. The digestion of the recombinant VWF occurs similar to the Furlan method. However, the breakdown of the multimers is assayed in a sandwich ELISA. First, the mixture is pipetted at 7 geometric dilutions of 1:20 to 1:1,024 into a microtiter plate the wells of which are coated with a monoclonal antibody (MoAB 454) to the C-terminal portion of VWF (AS 1366-2050). The second 125I-labeled antibody (a pool of monoclonal antibodies) is directed against the N-terminal portion of VWF. This means that the bound radioactivity is higher the less the VWF has been digested. In order to determine the activity of the protease, the dilution curve is used to determine the concentration at which 50% of the radioactivity is bound and

| Authors | Substrate | Denaturing | Incubation period | Method | Detection of protease action |
|---|---|---|---|---|---|
| Furlan et al. | Purified VWF | 1.5 m/L urea | Overnight | SDS-agarose gel electrophoresis, immune blot | Size of multimers |
| Tsai | Purified VWF | 0.15 m/L guanidine HCl | 1 hour | SDS-PAGE electrophoresis, immune blot | Occurrence of a 176 kd fragment (dimer) |
| Obert et al. | Recombinant VWF | 1.5 m/L urea | Overnight | 2-sided IRMA | Decrease in VWF:Ag |
| Gerritsen et al. | VWF in EDTA-treated/dialyzed plasma | 1.5 m/L urea | 2 hours | Residual VWF:CB | Decrease in VWF:CB |
| Böhm et al. | Purified VWF | 1.5 m/L urea | Overnight | Residual VWF:RCo | Decrease in VWF:RCo |
| Kokame et al. | Recombinant VWF fragment, VWF73 | None | 20-60 min | SDS-PAGE electrophoresis, immune blot | Occurrence of a proteolytic fragment |
| Whitelock et al. | A2 domain | None | 2 hours | ELISA | Decrease in the intact A2 domain |
| Zhou and Tsai | Recombinant VWF fragment, VWF73 | None | 3 hours | ELISA | Decrease in VWF73 |
| Kokame et al. | Recombinant VWF fragment, FRETS-VWF73 | None | 30-45 min | Fluorescence | Decrease in suppression of a fluorescent signal |

***Table 8.2:*** Published methods for assaying ADAMTS13 activity.

which binds a sample without protease activity (EDTA-treated sample). The dilution is compared with the dilution of a pool of normal plasma. Normal plasma is assigned an activity of 100%. Using this method, both the activity of ADAMTS13 and inhibitors of the protease are assayed. In a comparison test, values identical to Furlan's original method were obtained.

### 8.1.6. Rapid method by incubation of patient plasma in denaturing buffer

Here, endogenous VWF from patient plasma is used as the substrate. After incubation with, or dialysis in, denaturing Furlan buffer, the reaction is stopped by EDTA. The residual VWF:CB is then compared with that before dialysis, or electrophoretic demonstration of VWF multimers is undertaken. Although the latter is no longer a rapid method, demonstrating the multimers in fact shows the effect of the patient's ADAMTS13 on the patient's VWF.

### 8.1.7. FRETS assay

The smallest substrate that can still be effectively cleaved by ADAMTS13 extends for 73 amino acids from D1596 to R1668. In this substrate, Kokame et al. modified the amino acids Q1599 and N1610 so that they act as a fluorogen and quencher. The Y1605-M1606 bond can be cleaved by ADAMTS13, the quencher is thereby removed and there is fluorescence of the substrate (fluorescent resonance energy transfer, FRET). Using this substrate (FRETS-VWF73), the ADAMTS13 activity is assayed in a fluorimeter without denaturing substances. For the method to work optimally, however, unphysiological, low salt concentrations and activation by divalent cations ($Ca^{++}$) are also needed.

### 8.1.8. Method under conditions of a specific shear stress and in an endothelial cell-based system

Dong et al. developed a method that works under the more physiological conditions of a specific shear stress and on endothelial cells. Here, the supranormal multimers are proteolyzed in vivo directly on the surface of endothelial cells where the highest shear forces work. This test thus theoretically offers the possibility of detecting more defects than the test in the fluid phase, where binding to surfaces is not necessary. Endothelial cells are stimulated with histamine and then immobilized on the surface of a flow chamber with parallel plates. The plasma being studied is mixed with washed platelets and subjected to specific flow conditions in the chamber. The endothelial cells are then visually examined under the microscope. Without the addition of plasma, images resembling strings of pearls up to 3 mm long are seen, where the rows of "pearls" are platelets and the "string" consists of von Willebrand factor. This giant von Willebrand factor comes from the stimulated endothelial cells. After the addition of plasma, the strings very quickly disintegrate. As little as 5% plasma leads to a clear reduction in supranormal multimers within a few minutes. The test is quantitative under the described conditions and allows a calibration curve to be drawn between 6.25% and 50%. Patients with TTP may be diagnosed using this test. However, it remains to be proven whether using this method will allow detection of more cases of TTP with a severe reduction in protease than with the tests under static conditions.

### 8.1.9. Detection of non-neutralizing antibodies by an ELISA test

The above-described method for detecting neutralizing antibodies (inhibitors) fails in the presence of non-neutralizing antibodies. Moreover, it has been found to be not very sensitive and not very reliable. Scheiflinger et al. showed that a test for antibodies to ADAMTS13 is more sensitive than for the previously determined inhibitors and also detects non-neutralizing antibodies.

## 8.2. Molecular genetics

The specific VWF-cleaving protease was identified in 2001 to be a member of the ADAMTS family of metalloproteases and was called ADAMTS13 (A Disintegrin And Metalloproteinase with Thrombo-Spondin 1 like elements).

ADAMTS13 is located on the long arm of chromosome 9 (9q34). The genomic DNA measures 37 kb. The coding sequence consists of 29 exons with an open reading frame of 4,281 bp. cDNA analyses showed marked alternative splicing. It is thus possible that variants of the translation product have different functions and may perhaps be found in different tissues with a different frequency. The gene encodes a signal peptide of 33 amino acids and a propeptide of 41 amino acids, the actual metalloprotease domain, a disintegrin domain, a cysteine-rich domain with an RGDS sequence, a spacer and 8 thrombospondin-1-like motives as well as 2 so-called Cub domains, which are so far unique within the ADAMTS family (☞ Figure 8.3).

Three working groups characterized ADAMTS13 by pure isolation of the protease and peptide sequencing, while another working group localized the gene by linkage analysis of families with hereditary TTP and evidence of specific mutations of the ADAMTS13 gene. Since then, ADAMTS13 gene defects have been shown to be consistently responsible for the hereditary form of chronic recurrent TTP. In most cases, compound heterozygosity for ADAMTS13 mutations was found and only in a few consanguineous families homozygosity. This suggests marked heterogeneity of the mutation spectrum. The higher prevalence of missense mutations found in the initial study was interpreted to the effect that residual activity of the protease is essential for life. However, a further study found mainly nonsense and reading frame mutations, which were thought to correlate with a shortened or absent protein.

The mutation spectrum known today encompasses, apart from a high number of missense mutations, many truncating mutations and, in some instances, even mutations that are believed to be associated with complete absence of a functioning ADAMTS13 molecule. These include, for example, compound heterozygosity for a major ADAMTS13 deletion discovered by us and which includes exons 7 to 11 and a reading frame mutation (334delG) in exon 4 (☞ Figure 8.3, Table 8.3). This observation demonstrates that even complete ab-

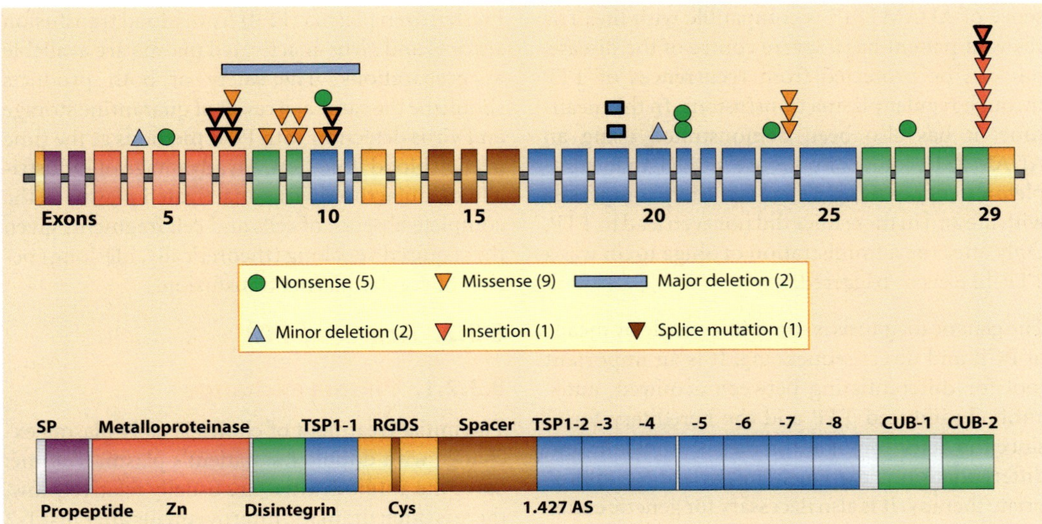


***Figure 8.3:*** Genomic and domain structure of ADAMTS13 based on Zheng et al. 2001, with the mutation spectrum of hereditary TTP in Germany and other European countries that we have recorded. Mutations of homozygous patients are outlined in bold.

| Patient | 1st mutation (nt) | 1st mutation (P) | Ex/In | 2nd mutation (nt) | 2nd mutation (P) | Ex/In |
|---|---|---|---|---|---|---|
| 1 | 334delG | frameshift | 4 | delExon7-11 | Deletion | 7 to 11 |
| 2 | 470G>A | W157X | 5 | 914A>G | Y305C | 8 |
| 3 | IVS6-2delA | Splice defect | In 6 | IVS6-2delA | Splice defect | In 6 |
| 4 | 695T>A | L232Q | 7 | 695T>A | L232Q | 7 |
| 5 | 788C>G | S263C | 7 | 4143insA | frameshift | 29 |
| 6 | 1022C>T | P341L | 9 | unknown | / | / |
| 7 | 1045C>T | R349C | 9 | 3107C>A | S1036X | 24 |
| 8 | 1058C>T | P353L | 9 | 2728C>T | R910X | 2 |
| 9 | 1058C>T | P353L | 9 | 4143insA | frameshift | 29 |
| 10 | 1169G>A | W390X | 10 | 2549-2550delAT | frameshift | 20 |
| 11 | 1170G>C | W390C | 10 | 3735G>A | W1245X | 27 |
| 12 | 1198T>C | C400R | 10 | 1198T>C | C400R | 10 |
| 13 | 2348del83 | Deletion | 19 | 2348del83 | Deletion | 19 |
| 14 | 2728C>T | R910X | 21 | 4143insA | frameshift | 29 |
| 15 | 3100A>T | R1034X | 24 | 4143insA | frameshift | 29 |
| 16 | 3178C>T | R1060W | 24 | 4143insA | frameshift | 29 |
| 17 | 3178C>T | R1060W | 24 | unknown | / | / |
| 18 | 3178C>T | R1060W | 24 | unknown | / | / |
| 19 | 4143insA | frameshift | 29 | 4143insA | frameshift | 29 |

***Table 8.3:*** Molecular genetic findings in the 19 patients with hereditary severe ADAMTS13 deficiency from Germany and other European countries that have so far been characterized in our laboratory. nt = nucleotide exchange, P = effect at protein level, Ex/In = localization in respective exon or intron. Due to autosomal recessive inheritance, the patients are either homozygous, or compound heterozygosity for 2 defects is to be expected. The identification of 2 mutations was not always possible.

sence of ADAMTS13 is compatible with life. The relevant patient has a severe course of the disease, but can be protected from recurrences of TTP through regular plasma transfusions. In the meantime, it has also been demonstrated using an ADAMTS13-knockout mouse model that complete absence of ADAMTS13 is entirely compatible with life and in these mice did not even lead to TTP. Only after the administration of Shiga toxin was a TTP-like event triggered.

The genetic diagnosis is sometimes made by means of PCR and direct sequencing. It is an important tool for differentiating between acquired, autoantibody-induced TTP and the hereditary form, since the detection of antibodies is unreliable and differentiation is extremely important for appropriate therapy. It is also necessary for genetic counseling.

## 8.3. Treatment

Before the observation that blood plasma had an effect in patients with TTP, more than 90% of patients died within a few days. However, in most cases, plasma infusion alone was not sufficient. Only daily plasma exchange over a sufficiently long period of time led to a breakthrough. At the current time, the mortality is about 10-20% and still very high, but has dramatically fallen compared with the era before plasma exchange. Most patients who require repeated plasma exchange generally have an antibody-mediated TTP. Only in the hereditary form is plasma infusion sufficient.

### 8.3.1. Hereditary TTP

In rare congenital deficiency of ADAMTS13, regular plasma infusion is sufficient. Fortunately, the protease has a relatively long half-life of about 3 days. Thus, infusion of plasma every 1-2 weeks is sufficient in patients who are chronically thrombocytopenic without regular administration of protease and experience life-threatening crises in acute situations. The infusion interval can be very easily established based on the behavior of the platelet count. Alloantibodies to the protease have not so far been described; however, alloantibodies are theoretically to be expected if the patients do not produce any protease themselves (foreign protein).

Fresh frozen plasma (FFP) from blood transfusion services and virus-inactivated plasma are available as preparations. The safety of both products should be the same as a result of quarantine storage and virus detection with PCR methods at the time of each blood donation. An advantage of industrially manufactured virus-inactivated plasma is the complete absence of cells and cell fragments given the required very long (theoretically, life-long) period of regular plasma transfusions.

### 8.3.2. Acquired TTP

#### 8.3.2.1. Plasma exchange

The initial treatment of choice is daily plasma exchange with double the patient's plasma volume. Since the antibody titers are usually relatively low, there is often dramatic improvements after just 1-2 days. However, the antibody is frequently boostered as a result of this and there is a period during which the patients can survive only with exchange therapy over many days or even weeks. Some of the patients subsequently lose the antibody and do not have a recurrence. In an initial clinical remission, but with persistent antibodies, there is the danger that regularly recurring TTP develops. These patients have only short phases of remission and must be very rapidly retreated. Other patients have recurrences much less commonly but develop recurrence again every 1-2 years. These patients usually have no detectable antibody in the intervening period.

#### 8.3.2.2. Immunosuppression/immunomodulation

Even before the discovery of ADAMTS13 and ADAMTS13 antibodies, virtually all patients additionally received corticosteroids. This clinical practice was retrospectively shown to be clearly indicated. If cortisone was not sufficiently immunosuppressant or had too many side effects, cyclophosphamide was administered in addition, usually with only little success. Vinca alcaloids not only have an immunosuppressant effect but also interfere with the functional capability of the platelets. They destroy the microtubules of the circulating platelets and thereby prevent adhesion and aggregation of these. In emergency situations, rapid successes can be achieved as a result of this. However, as soon as fresh platelets reach the circulation, this effect is lost.

#### 8.3.2.3. Splenectomy

Splenectomy has proven useful in patients who were refractory to all of the above therapeutic measures. It can usually be undertaken without any problems even in the presence of low platelet counts and in nearly all reported cases leads to lasting remission. In a female patient with antibody-induced TTP whom we treated, a normal ADAMTS13 could not be detected for nearly a year despite a prompt clinical remission. After a few months, the antibody initially disappeared then the protease slowly increased to be within the low normal range. From activity of 18%, schistocytes and supranormal multimers were visible without the blood count being pathological. In the presence of residual activity of 10%, a prominent feature was mild anemia, the schistocytes could no longer be overlooked and there were marked supranormal multimers. At the current time, the patient is in remission with stable ADAMTS13 levels of about 25% This is probably her normal protease activity, since she is heterozygous for a causal ADAMTS13 mutation (R1060W).

#### 8.3.2.4. Antibodies to B cells

Rituximab, an anti-CD20 antibody, was developed for the treatment of patients with multiple myeloma and B-cell lymphoma. After standard therapy that normally involves four administrations of the drug, B cells can no longer be detected. Since antibody-producing cells are also eliminated as a result, this treatment represents a fascinating possibility for achieving remission in refractory cases of TTP. The first German patient is a small boy who has had a disease course with many severe complications over several years and has been in stable remission since. The cases reported in the literature and the 26 patients in Germany known to us because of follow-up assays nearly all benefit from this treatment and achieve stable remissions. However, here too treatment failure rates of 10-20% may be expected. There are no data on the length of remission since the treatment only started to be used a few years ago. A noticeable feature here again is that the clinical remission precedes normal ADAMTS13 levels by many months.

#### 8.3.2.5. Treatment with antiplatelet agents

Acetylsalicylic acid (ASA) has no place in primary therapy because of the often severe thrombocytopenia. It has been, and continues to be, frequently used for prophylaxis in phases of remission. To date, this treatment has not been shown to be successful. There are even fewer reliable data for clopidogrel than for ASS. Drugs that inhibit the GP IIb/IIIa receptor are much more effective than ASS and clopidogrel. However, they interfere with the wrong receptor and cannot inhibit the initial reaction between platelets and VWF that occurs via the GP Ib/IX complex. Thus, these drugs do not currently have a reliable place in the treatment of TTP either.

#### 8.3.2.6. TTP after bone marrow transplantation

This complication may be expected in about 15 % of patients after bone marrow transplantations. ADAMTS13 falls to low levels but rarely goes below 10%. The success of treatment with infusion of plasma or a plasma exchange is rather moderate. A definite therapeutic recommendation is not yet possible.

#### 8.3.2.7. TTP in malignant diseases

There are no clear findings here either. A definite therapeutic recommendation cannot therefore be made.

#### 8.3.2.8. Drug-induced TTP

About 50 different drugs are suspected of causing microangiopathic thrombocytopenia. In most cases, however, HUS is observed.

A typical form of TTP is caused by ticlopidine, and more rarely clopidogrel. In most cases, an antibody to the protease is induced. Cases without demonstrable antibodies but greatly reduced protease are also known with clopidogrel. The initially high mortality has been greatly reduced as a result of treatment with plasma exchange.

Patients who experience severe, usually fatal microangiopathic disease while in remission from tumor disease after treatment with mitomycin or other cytostatics usually present with HUS, rarely with the clinical picture of TTP. According to literature reports, immune adsorption considerably improves the prognosis of these patients. Life-threatening complications typically occur with blood transfusions. These should thus be kept to a minimum.

Vincristine is used for the treatment of TTP, but in very rare cases may also trigger this condition. The treatment is not different from that of antibody-induced TTP.

# References

# 9. References


## 1. History

von Willebrand EA. Hereditär pseudohemofili. Finska Läk Sällsk Handl, 68: 87-112, 1926

von Willebrand E A, Jürgens R. Über ein neues vererbbares Blutungsübel: die konstitutionelle Thrombopathie. Dtsch Arch Klin Med, 175: 453-483, 1933

Kehrer FA. Die Hämophilie beim weiblichen Geschlecht. Arch Gynäkol, 10:14-237, 1876

Alexander B, Goldstein R. Dual hemostatic defect in pseudohemophilia. J Clin Invest 32: 551-557, 1953

Nilsson IM, Blombäck M, von Francken I. On an inherited autosomal hemorrhagic diathesis with antihemophilic globulin (AHG) deficiency and prolonged bleeding time. Acta Med Scand 159: 53-57, 1957

Zimmerman TS, Ratnoff OD, Powell AE. Immunologic differentiation of classic hemophilia (factor VIII deficiency) and von Willebrand's disease, with observations on combined deficiencies of antihemophilic factor and proaccelerin (factor V) and on an acquired circulating anticoagulant against antihemophilic factor. J Clin Invest, 50: 244-254, 1971

Mancuso DJ, Tuley EA, Westfield LA et al. Structure of the gene for human von Willebrand factor. J Biol Chem, 264: 19514-15927, 1989

Mancuso DJ, Tuley EA, Westfield LA et al. Human von Willebrand factor gene and pdeudogene: Structural analysis and differentiation by polymerase chain reaction. Biochemistry, 30: 253-269, 1991

## 2. Clinical Symptoms and Genetics

Rodeghiero F, Castaman G. Congenital von Willebrand disease type I: definition, phenotypes, clinical and laboratory assesment. Bailliere´s Clinical Haematology, 14: 321-335, 2001

DiPaola J, Federici AB, Mannucci PM et al. Low platelet alpha(2)beta(1) levels in type 1 von Willebrand disease correlate with impaired platelet function in a high shear stress system. Blood, 93: 3578-3582, 1999

Cornu P, Larrieu MJ, Caen J et al. Transfusion studies in von Willebrand disease: effect on bleeding time and factor. VIII, Br J Haematol 1963; 9: 189–202.

Ginsburg D, Konkle BA, Gill JC, Montgomery RR, Bockenstedt PL, Johnson TA & Yang AY. Molecular basis of human von Willebrand disease: analysis of platelet von Willebrand factor mRNA. Proc Natl Acad Sci USA 1989;86: 3723-3727

## 3. von Willebrand Factor (VWF)

de Wit TR, van Mourik JA. Biosynthesis, processing and secretion of von Willebrand factor: biological implications. Bailliere´s Clinical Haematology, 14: 241-255, 2001

Ruggeri ZM. Structure of von Willebrand factor and its function in platelet adhesion and thrombus formation. Bailliere´s Clinical Haematology, 14: 257-278, 2001

Schneppenheim R, Budde U, Obser T et al. Expression and characterization of von Willebrand dimerization defects in different types of von Willebrand disease. Blood, 97: 2059-2066, 2001

Schneppenheim R, Brassard J, Krey S, Budde U, Kunicki TJ, Holmerg L, Ware J, Ruggeri ZM. Defective dimerization of von Willebrand factor subunits due to a Cys Arg mutation in IID von Willebrand disease. Proc Natl Acad Sci U.S.A., 938: 3581-3586, 1996

Gaucher C, Dieval J, Mazurier C. Characterization of von Willebrand factor gene defects in two unrelated patients with type IIC von Willebrand disease. Blood, 84: 1024-1030, 1994

Schneppenheim R, Thomas KB, Krey S, Budde U, Jessat U, Sutor AH, Zieger B. Identification of a candidate missense mutation in a family with von Willebrand disease type IIC. Human Genetics, 956: 681-686, 1995

Furlan M, Robles R, Solenthaler M, Lämmle B. Acquired deficiency of von Willebrand factor-cleaving protease in a patient with thrombotic thrombocytopenic purpura. Blood, 91: 3097-3103, 1997

Schneppenheim R, Krey S, Bergmann F, Bock D, Budde U, Lange M, Linde R, Mittler U, Meili E, Mertes G, Olek K, Plendl H, Simeoni E. Genetic heterogeneity of severe von Willebrand disease type III in the German population. Human Genet 94: 640-652, 1994

Meyer D, Fressinaud E, Hilbert L, Ribba A, Lavergne JM, Mazurier C. Type 2 von Willebrand disease causing defective von Willebrand factor-dependent platelet function. Bailliere´s Clinical Haematology, 14: 349-364, 2001

Michiels JJ (ed.). Von Willebrand factor and von Willebrand disease. Baillieres Best Pract Res. Clin Haematol, 14: 235-462, 2001

Schneppenheim R, Budde U. Phenotypic and genotypic diagnosis of von Willebrand disease: a 2004 update. Semin Hematol. 2005;42:15-28

Dopheide SM, Maxwell MJ, Jackson SP. Shear-dependent tether fomation during platelet transduction on von Willebrand factor. Blood, 99: 159-167, 2002

Kunicki, TJ. Gene regulation of platelet function. In: Platelets in thrombotic and non-thrombotic disorders.

Eds. Gresle P, Page CP, Fuster V, Vermylen J. Cambridge University Press pp 760-779

Mazurier C. Von Willebrand disease masquerading as haemophilia A. Thromb Haemost, 67: 391-396, 1992

## 4. Classification and Pathogenesis

Rugggeri ZM. Classification of von Willebrand disease. In: Thrombosis and Haemostasis 1987. Ed. Verstraete M, Vermylen J, Lijnen R and Arnout J. Leuven: Leuven University Press, pp 419-445.

Sadler JE, Budde U, Eikenboom JC, Favaloro EJ, Hill FG, Holmberg L, Ingerslev J, Lee CA, Lillicrap D, Mannucci PM, Mazurier C, Meyer D, Nichols WL, Nishino M, Peake IR, Rodeghiero F, Schneppenheim R, Ruggeri ZM, Srivastava A, Montgomery RR, Federici AB; the Working Party on von Willebrand Disease Classification. Update on the pathophysiology and classification of von Willebrand disease: a report of the Subcommittee on von Willebrand Factor. J Thromb Haemost. 4: 2103-2114, 2006.

Sadler EJ, Gralnick HR. Commentary: A new classification for von Willebrand disease. Blood, 84: 676-679, 1994.

Schneppenheim R, Budde U, Ruggeri ZM. A molecular approach to the classification of von Willebrand disease. Bailliere´s Clinical Haematology, 14: 281-298, 2001.

## 5. Diagnosis

Rodeghiero F, Castaman GC, Dini E. Epidemiological investigation of the prevalence of von Willebrand's disease. Blood: 69: 454-459, 1987.

Werner EJ, Emmett H, Tucker E, Giroux D, Schultz J, Abshire T. Prevalence of von Willebrand disease in children. A multiethnic study. J Pediatr 123: 93-98, 1993.

Budde U, Drewke E, Mainusch K, Schneppenheim R. Laboratory diagnosis of congenital von Willebrand disease. Sem Thromb Haemost 28: 173-189, 2002

Ruggeri ZM, Zimmerman TS. Variant von Willebrand's disease. Characterization of two subtypes by analysis of multimeric composition of factor VIII/von Willebrand factor in plasma and platelets. J Clin Invest, 65: 1318-1325, 1980.

Dent JA, Galbusera M, Ruggeri ZM. Heterogeneity of plasma von Willebrand factor multimers resulting from proteolysis of the constituent subunit. J Clin Invest, 88: 774-782

Duke WW. The relation of blood platelets to hemorrhagic disease. JAMA, 55: 1185-1192, 1910.

Ivy AC, Shapiro PF, Melnick P. The bleeding tendency in jaundice. Surg Gynecol Obstet, 60: 781-784, 1935.

Fressinaud E, Veyradier A, Truchaud F et al. Screening for von Willebrand disease with a new analyzer using high shear stress: A study of 60 cases. Blood, 91: 1232-1231, 1998.

Hubbard AR, Rigsby P, Barrowcliffe TW. Standardisation of factor VIII and von Willebrand factor in plasma: Calibration of the 4th International Standard (97/586). Thromb Haemost, 85: 634-638, 2001.

Gralnick HR, Rick ME, McKeown LP. Platelet von Willebrand factor: An important determinant of the bleeding time in type I von Willebrand's disease. Blood, 68: 58-61, 1986.

Cejka J. Enzyme immunoassay for factor VIII-related antigen. Clin Chem, 28: 1356-1358, 1992.

Veyradier A, Fressinaud E, Sigaud M, Wolf M, Meyer D. A new automated method for von Willebrand factor antigen measurement using latex particles. Thromb Haemost, 81: 320-321, 1999.

Weiss HJ, Hoyer LW, Rickles F, Varma A, Rogers J. Quantitative assay of a plasma factor in von Willebrand's disease that is necessary for platelet aggregation. J Clin Invest, 52: 2701-2716, 1973.

Brown JE, Bosak JO. An ELISA test for the binding of von Willebrand factor antigen to collagen. Thromb Res, 43: 303-311, 1986.

Schneppenheim R, Plendl H, Budde U. Luminography - an alternative assay for detection of von Willebrand factor multimers. Thromb Haemost, 60:133-136,1988.

Mazurier C, Goudemand J, Hilbert L, Caron C, Fressinaud E, Meyer D. Type 2N von Willebrand disease: clinical maniestations, pathophysiology, laboratory diagnosis and molecular biology. Bailliere´s Clinical Haematology, 14: 337-347, 2001.

Ginburg D, Konkle BA, Gill JC et al. Molecular basis of human von Willebrand disease: analysis of platelet von Willebrand factor mRNA. Proc Natl Acad Sci U.S.A., 86: 3723-3727, 1989.

Schneppenheim R, Obser T, Schneppenheim S, Mainusch K, Angerhaus D, Budde U. Von Willebrand disease type 2A with aberrant structure of individual oligomers is caused by mutations clustering in the von Willebrand factor D3 domain. Blood, 96: 566a, 2000 (abstr.).

Ledford M, Rabinowtz I, Sadler JE et al. New variant of von Willebrand disease type II with markedly increased levels of von Willebrand factor antigen and dominant mode of inheritance: von Willebrand disease type IIC Miami. Blood, 82: 169-175, 1993.

Weiss HJ, Sussman II. A new von Willebrand variant (type I, New York): increased ristocetin-induced platelet aggregation and plasma von Willebrand factor containing the full range of multimers. Blood, 68: 149-156, 1986.

Ware J, Dent JA, Azuma H. Identification of point mutations in type IIB von Willebrand disease illustrating the regulation of von Willebrand factor affinity for the platelet membrane glycoprotein Ib-IX receptor. Proc Natl Acad Sci U.S.A., 887: 2946-2950, 1991.

Schneppenheim R, Federici AB, Budde U et al. Von Willebrand disease type 2M "Vicenza" in Italian and German patients: identification of the first candidate mutation (G3864R; R1205H) in 8 families. Thromb Haemost, 83: 136-140, 2000.

Schneppenheim R, Budde U, Krey S et al. Results of a screening for von Willebrand disease type 2N patients with suspected haemophilia A or von Willebrand disease type 1. Thromb Haemost, 76: 598-602, 1996

## 6. Acquired von Willebrand Disease

Simone JV, Cornet JA, Abildgaard CF: Acquired von Willebrand's syndrome in systemic lupus erythematodes. Blood 31: 806-811,1968

Ingram GIC, Kingston PJ, Leslie J, Bowie EJW. Four cases of acquired von Willebrand's syndrome. Br J Haematol 21: 189-191, 1971

Mant MJ, Gauldie HJ, Bienestock GJ, Pineo GF, Luke KH. Von Willebrand's syndrome presenting as an acquired bleeding disorder in association with a monoclonal gammapathy. Blood 42: 429-436, 1973

Budde U, Schäfer G, Müller N, Egli H, Dent J, Ruggeri ZM, Zimmerman TS. Acquired von Willebrand's disease in the myeloproliferative syndrome. Blood 64: 981-985, 1984

Budde U, Dent J, Berkowitz SD, Ruggeri ZM, Zimmermann TS: Subunit composition of plasma von Willebrand factor in patients with the myeloproliferative syndrome. Blood 68: 1213-1217, 1986

Gill JC, Wilson AD, Endres-Brooks J, Montgomery RR. Loss of the largest von Willebrand factor multimers from plasma of patients with congenital cardiac defects. Blood 67: 758-761, 1986

Kinoshita S, Yoshioka K, Kasahara M, Takamiya O. Acquired von Willebrand disease after Epstein-Barr virus infection. J Pediatr 1119: 595-598, 1991

Jakway JL. Acquired von Willebrand's disease in malignancy. Sem Thromb Hemost 18: 434-439, 1992

Rinder MR, Richard RE, Rinder HM. Acquired von Willebrand's disease: a concise review. Am J Hematol 54: 139-145, 1997

Tefferi A, Nichols WL. Acquired von Willebrand disease: concise review of occurrence, diagnosis, pathogenesis and treatment. Am J Med 103: 536-540, 1997

Michiels JJ, Budde U, van Genderen PJJ, van der Planken M, van Vliet HHDM, Schroyens W, Berneman Z. Acquired von Willebrand Syndromes: Clinical features, etiology, pathophysiology, classification and management. Baillère's Clinical Haematology 14: 401-436, 2001

Veyradier A, Jenkins CSP, Fressinaud E, Meyer D. Acquired von Willebrand syndrome: From pathophysiology to management. Thromb Haemost 84: 175-182, 2000

Federici AB, Rand JH, Bucciarelli P, Budde U, van Genderen PJJ, Mohri H, Meyer D, Rodeghiero F, Sadler E. Acquired von Willebrand syndrome: Data from an international registry. Thromb Haemost 84: 345-349, 2000

Luboshitz J, Lubetsky A, Schliamser L, Kotler A, Tamarin I, Inbal A. Pharmacokinetic studies with FVIII/von Willebrand factor concentrate can be a diagnostic tool to distinguish between subgroups of patients with acquired von Willebrand syndrome. Thromb Haemost 85: 806-809, 2001

Van Genderen PJJ, Terpstra W, Michiels JJ, Kapteijn L, van Vliet HHDM. High-dose intravenous immunoglobulin delays clearance of von Willebrand factor in acquired von Willebrand disease. Throm Haemost 73: 891-892, 1995

Budde U, Scharf RE, Franke P, Hartmann-Budde K, Dent J, Ruggeri ZM. Elevated platelet count as a cause of abnormal von Willebrand factor multimer distribution in plasma. Blood 82: 749-1757, 1993

Van Genderen PJJ, Budde U, Michiels JJ, van Strik R, van Vliet HHDM. The reduction of large von Willebrand factor multimers in patients with essential thrombocythemia is related to the platelet count. Br J Haematol 93: 962-965, 1996.

Knobloch W, Hauser E, Niehues R, Schiele T, Metzger G, Jacksch R. Calcifying aortic valve stenosis and cryptogenic gastrointestinal bleeding (Heyde syndrome): report of two cases. Zeitschr Kardiol 88: 448-453, 1999

Pareti FI, Lattuada A, Bressi C, Zanobini M, Sala A, Steffan A, Ruggeri ZM. Proteolysis of von Willebrand factor and shear stress-induced platelet aggregation in patients with aortic valve stenosis. Circulation 102: 1290-1295, 2000

Heyde EC. Gastrointestinal bleeding in aortic stenosis. N Engl J Med 259: 196, 1958 (letter)

Warkentin TE, Moore JC, Morgan DG. Aortic stenosis and bleeding gastrointestinal angiodysplasia - Is acquired von Willebrands disease the link? Lancet 340: 35-37, 1992

Kreuz W, Linde R, Funk M, Meyer Schrod R, Foll E, Nowak Göttl U, Jacobi G, Vigh Z, Scharrer I. Induction of von Willebrand disease type 1 by valproic acid. Lancet 335: 178-1350, 1990

Gralnick HR, McKeown LP, Willimas SB, Shafer BC. Plasma and platelet von Willebrand factor: defects in uremia. Am J Med 85: 806-810, 1988

Dentale N, Fulgaro C, Guerra L, Fasulo G, Mazzetti M, Fabbri C. Acquisition of factor VIII inhibitor after acute hepatitis C virus infection. Blood 90: 3233-3234, 1997

Budde U, Bergmann F, Michiels JJ. Acquired von Willebrand syndrome: Experience from 2 years in a single laboratory compared with data from the literature and an international registry. Sem Thromb Haemost 28: 277-237, 2002

Mannucci PM, Ruggeri ZM, Pareti FI, Capitanio A. D.D.A.V.P. in haemophilia. Lancet 2:1171-1172, 1977

Mannucci PM. How I treat patients with von Willebrand disease. Blood 97:1915-1919, 2001

Federici AB, Mazurier C, Berntorp E, Lee CA, Scharrer I, Goudemand J, Lethagen S, Nitu I, Ludwig G, Hilbert L, Mannucci PM. Related Articles, Links Abstract Biological response to desmopressin in patients with severe type 1 and type 2 von Willebrand disease: results of a multicenter European study. Blood 103: 2032-2038, 2004.

## 7. Treatment of von Willebrand Disease

Mannucci PM, Ruggeri ZM, Pareti FI, Capitanio A. D.D.A.V.P. in haemophilia. Lancet 1977; ii:1171-1172, 1977

Mannucci PM. Desmopressin (DDAVP) in the treatment of bleeding disorders. The first 20 years. Blood 1997;90:2515-2521

Federici AB, Mazurier C, Berntorp E, Lee CA, Scharrer I, Goudemand J, Lethagen S, Nitu I, Ludwig G, Hilbert L, Mannucci PM. Biologic response to desmopressin in patients with severe type 1 and type 2 von Willebrand disease: Results of a multicenter European study. Blood 2004;103:2032-2038

Castaman G, Rodeghiero F. Desmopressin and type IIB von Willebrand disease. Hemophilia 1996; 2: 73-76

Castaman G, Lethagen S, Federici AB, Tosetto A, Goodeve A, Budde U, Battle J, Meyer D, Mazurier C, Fressinaud E, Goudemand J, Eikenboom J, Schneppenheim R, Ingerslev J, Vorlova Z, Habart D, Holmberg L, Pasi J, Hill F, Peake I, Rodeghiero F. Response of desmopressin influenced by the genotype and phenotype in type 1 von Willebrand disease: results from the European study MCMDM-1VWD. Blood 2008; 111: 3531-3539

Nichols WL, Hultin MB, James AH, Manco-Johnson MJ, Montgomery RR, Ortel TL, Rick ME, Sadler JE, Weinstein M, Yawn BP. Von willebrand disease (VWD): evidence-based diagnosis and management guidelines, the National Heart, Lung, and blood Institute (NHLBI) Expert Panel report (USA). Haemophilia 2008; 14: 171-232.

Michiels JJ, Budde U, van Genderen PJJ, van der Planken M, van Vliet HHDM, Schroyens W, Berneman Z. Acquired von Willebrand Syndromes: Clinical features, etiology, pathophysiology, classification and management. Baillère's Clinical Haematology 2001;14:401-436

## 8. Thrombotic Thrombocytopenic Purpura (TTP)

Moschcowitz E. Hyaline thrombosis of the terminal arterioles and capillaries: a hitherto undescribed disease. Proc N Y Pathol Soc 24: 21-24, 1924

Schulman I, Pierce M, Lukens A, Currimbhoy Z. Studies on thrombopoiesis. I. A factor in normal human plasma required for platelet production; chronic thrombocytopenia due to its deficiency. Blood 16: 943-957, 1960

Upshaw JD Jr. Congenital deficiency of a factor in normal plasma that reverses microangiopathic hemolysis and thrombocytopenia. N Engl J Med 298: 1350-1352, 1978

Moake JL, Rudy CK, Troll JH, Weinstein MJ, Colannino NM, Azocar J, Seder RH, Hong SL, Deykin D. Unusually large plasma factor VIII:von Willebrand factor multimers in chronic relapsing thrombotic thrombocytopenic purpura. N Engl J Med 307: 1432-1435, 1982

Furlan M, Robles R, Lämmle B. Partial purification and characterization of a protease from human plasma cleaving von Willebrand factor to fragments produced by in vivo proteolysis. Blood 87: 4223-4234, 1996

Tsai HM. Physiologic cleavage of von Willebrand factor by a plasma protease is dependent on its conformation and requires calcium ion. Blood 87: 4235-4244,1996

Furlan M, Robles R, Galbusera M, Remuzzi G, Kyrle PA, Brenner B, Krause M, Scharrer I, Aumann V, Mittler U, Solenthaler M, Lammle B. von Willebrand factor-cleaving protease in thrombotic thrombocytopenic purpura and the hemolytic-uremic syndrome. N Engl J Med 339: 1578-1584, 1998

Gerritsen HE, Turecek PL, Schwarz HP, Lämmle B, Furlan M. Assay of von Willebrand factor (VWF)-cleaving protease based on decreased collagen binding affinity of degraded VWF: a tool for the diagnosis of thrombotic thrombocytopenic purpura (TTP) Thromb Haemost 82: 1386-1389, 1999

Kokame K, Nobe Y, Kokubo Y, Okayama A, Miyata T. FRETS-VWF73, a first fluorogenic substrate for ADAMTS13 assay. Br J Haematol. 2005;129:93-100

Fujikawa K, Suzuki H, McMullen B, Chung D. Purification of human von Willebrand factor-cleaving protease and its identification as a new member of the metalloproteinase family. Blood 98: 1662-1666, 2001

Zheng X, Chung D, Takayama TK, Majerus EM, Sadler JE, Fujikawa K. Structure of von Willebrand factor-cleaving protease (ADAMTS13), a metalloprotease involved in thrombotic thrombocytopenic purpura. J Biol Chem 276: 41059-41063, 2001

Levy GG, Nichols WC, Lian EC, Foroud T, McClintick JN, McGee BM, Yang AY, Siemieniak DR, Stark KR, Gruppo R, Sarode R, Shurin SB, Chandrasekaran V, Stabler SP, Sabio H, Bouhassira EE, Upshaw JD Jr, Ginsburg D, Tsai HM. Mutations in a member of the ADAMTS gene family cause thrombotic thrombocytopenic purpura. Nature 413: 488-494, 2001

Schneppenheim R, Budde U, Oyen F et al. Von Willebrand factor cleaving protease and ADAMTS13 mutations in childhood TTP. Blood 101: 1845-1850, 2002

Schneppenheim R, Budde U, Hassenpflug W, Obser T. Severe ADAMTS-13 deficiency in childhood. Semin Hematol. 2004; 41:83-89

Budde U, Angerhaus D, Obser T, Schneppenheim R. Diagnose der Thrombotisch Thrombozytopenischen Purpura, Hämostaseologie. 2004;24:65-70

Chauhan AK, Kisucka J, Brill A, Walsh MT, Scheiflinger F, Wagner DD. ADAMTS13: a new link between thrombosis and inflammation. J Exp Med. 2008 Sep 1;205:2065-74

Chauhan AK, Motto DG, Lamb CB, Bergmeier W, Dockal M, Plaimauer B, Scheiflinger F, Ginsburg D, Wagner DD. Systemic antithrombotic effects of ADAMTS13. J Exp Med. 2006;203:767-76

# Index

# Index

## A



## B



## C



## D



## E



## F



## G



## H



## I



## L



## M



## N



## O



## P

## R



## S



## T



## U



## V



## W

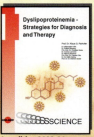

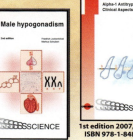